T0073707

Access your Clinics anywhere you go with our new App!

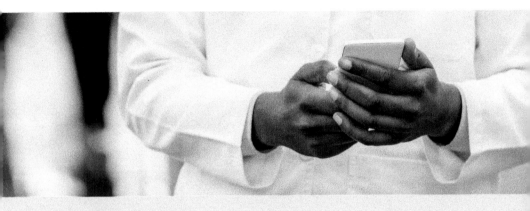

The new and improved Clinics Review Articles mobile app offers subscribers rapid access to recently published content from all Clinics Review Articles titles.

KEY FEATURES OF THE CLINICS APP:

- **Download full issues** while reading – no need to wait!
- **Access articles quickly and conveniently** with new, improved layouts and navigation.
- **Interact with figures, tables, videos**, and other supplementary content.
- **Personalize your experience** by creating reading lists and adding your own notes to articles.
- **Share your favorite articles** on social media and email useful content to colleagues.

DOWNLOAD THE CLINICS APP TODAY!

Clinics Review Articles

Perinatal Mental Health

Editors

CONSTANCE GUILLE
ROGER B. NEWMAN

OBSTETRICS AND GYNECOLOGY CLINICS OF NORTH AMERICA

www.obgyn.theclinics.com

Consulting Editor
WILLIAM F. RAYBURN

September 2018 • Volume 45 • Number 3

ELSEVIER

1600 John F. Kennedy Boulevard • Suite 1800 • Philadelphia, Pennsylvania, 19103-2899

http://www.theclinics.com

OBSTETRICS AND GYNECOLOGY CLINICS OF NORTH AMERICA Volume 45, Number 3
September 2018 ISSN 0889-8545, ISBN-13: 978-0-323-64229-3

Editor: Kerry Holland
Developmental Editor: Kristen Helm

Obstetrics and Gynecology Clinics (ISSN 0889-8545) is published quarterly by Elsevier Inc., 360 Park Avenue South, New York, NY 10010-1710. Months of issue are March, June, September, and December. Periodicals postage paid at New York, NY, and additional mailing offices. Subscription price per year is $313.00 (US individuals), $652.00 (US institutions), $100.00 (US students), $393.00 (Canadian individuals), $823.00 (Canadian institutions), $225.00 (Canadian students), $459.00 (international individuals), $823.00 (international institutions), and $225.00 (international students). To receive student/resident rate, orders must be accompanied by name of affiliated institution, date of term, and the signature of program/residency coordinator on institution letterhead. Orders will be billed at individual rate until proof of status is received. Foreign air speed delivery is included in all *Clinics* subscription prices. All prices are subject to change without notice. POSTMASTER: Send address changes to *Obstetrics and Gynecology Clinics*, Elsevier Health Sciences Division, Subscription Customer Service, 3251 Riverport Lane, Maryland Heights, MO 63043. **Customer Service: Telephone: 1-800-654-2452 (U.S. and Canada); 314-447-8871 (outside U.S. and Canada). Fax: 314-447-8029. E-mail: journalscustomerservice-usa@elsevier.com (for print support); journalsonlinesupport-usa@elsevier.com (for online support).**

Reprints. For copies of 100 or more of articles in this publication, please contact the Commercial Reprints Department, Elsevier Inc., 360 Park Avenue South, New York, New York 10010-1710. Tel.: 212-633-3874; Fax: 212-633-3820; E-mail: reprints@elsevier.com.

Obstetrics and Gynecology Clinics of North America is also published in Spanish by McGraw-Hill Interamericana Editores S.A., P.O. Box 5-237, 06500, Mexico; in Portuguese by Reichmann and Affonso Editores, Rio de Janeiro, Brazil; and in Greek by Paschalidis Medical Publications, Athens, Greece.

Obstetrics and Gynecology Clinics of North America is covered in *MEDLINE/PubMed (Index Medicus), Excerpta Medica, Current Concepts/Clinical Medicine, Science Citation Index, BIOSIS, CINAHL,* and *ISI/BIOMED.*

Printed in the United States of America.

Contributors

CONSULTING EDITOR

WILLIAM F. RAYBURN, MD, MBA
Associate Dean, Continuing Medical Education and Professional Development, Distinguished Professor and Emeritus Chair, Obstetrics and Gynecology, University of New Mexico School of Medicine, Albuquerque, New Mexico

EDITORS

CONSTANCE GUILLE, MD, MSCR
Director, Women's Reproductive Behavioral Health Program, Associate Professor, Departments of Psychiatry and Behavioral Sciences, and Obstetrics and Gynecology, Medical University of South Carolina, Charleston, South Carolina

ROGER B. NEWMAN, MD
Professor and Maas Endowed Chair for Reproductive Sciences, Department of Obstetrics and Gynecology, Medical University of South Carolina, Charleston, South Carolina

AUTHORS

ROSAURA ORENGO AGUAYO, PhD
Assistant Professor, Department of Psychiatry and Behavioral Sciences, Medical University of South Carolina, National Crime Victims Research and Treatment Center (NCVRTC), Charleston, South Carolina

ALLISON S. BAKER, MD
Instructor of Psychiatry, Psychiatrist, Perinatal and Reproductive Psychiatry Program, Harvard Medical School, Massachusetts General Hospital, Boston, Massachusetts

CYNTHIA L. BATTLE, PhD
Associate Professor, Department of Psychiatry and Human Behavior, The Warren Alpert Medical School of Brown University, Associate Director, Psychosocial Research Program, Butler Hospital, Research Psychologist, Center for Women's Behavioral Health, Women & Infants Hospital of Rhode Island, Providence, Rhode Island

LISA BOYARS, MD
Assistant Professor, Department of Psychiatry and Behavioral Sciences, Medical University of South Carolina, Charleston, South Carolina

TONIA M. CASSADAY, MSW, LISW-CP/S
Clinical Instructor, Department of Psychiatry, Medical University of South Carolina, North Charleston, South Carolina

CRYSTAL T. CLARK, MD, MSc
Assistant Professor of Psychiatry and Behavioral Sciences and Obstetrics and Gynecology, Northwestern University Feinberg School of Medicine, Chicago, Illinois

ELIZABETH COX, MD
Assistant Professor, Department of Psychiatry, The University of North Carolina at Chapel Hill, Chapel Hill, North Carolina

KRISTINA M. DELIGIANNIDIS, MD
Director, Women's Behavioral Health, Zucker Hillside Hospital, Northwell Health, Glen Oaks, New York; Associate Professor, Departments of Psychiatry and Obstetrics and Gynecology, Donald and Barbara Zucker School of Medicine at Hofstra/Northwell, Hempstead, New York; Feinstein Institute for Medical Research, Manhasset, New York

ELIZABETH H. EUSTIS, MA
Psychology Resident, Department of Psychiatry and Human Behavior, The Warren Alpert Medical School of Brown University, Providence, Rhode Island

PHYLLIS M. FLORIAN, PsyD
Prospicare, Kalamazoo, Michigan

MARLENE P. FREEMAN, MD
Associate Professor of Psychiatry, Associate Director, Perinatal and Reproductive Psychiatry Program, Harvard Medical School, Medical Director, CTNI, Abra Prentice Foundation Chair, Women's Mental Health, Massachusetts General Hospital, Boston, Massachusetts

EDITH GETTES, MD
Assistant Professor, Department of Psychiatry, The University of North Carolina at Chapel Hill, Chapel Hill, North Carolina

AMANDA K. GILMORE, PhD
Research Assistant Professor, Medical University of South Carolina, College of Nursing, Charleston, South Carolina

CONSTANCE GUILLE, MD, MSCR
Director, Women's Reproductive Behavioral Health Program, Associate Professor, Departments of Psychiatry and Behavioral Sciences, and Obstetrics and Gynecology, Medical University of South Carolina, Charleston, South Carolina

CHRISTINE K. HAHN, PhD
Postdoctoral Research Fellow, Department of Psychiatry and Behavioral Sciences, Medical University of South Carolina, National Crime Victims Research and Treatment Center (NCVRTC), Charleston, South Carolina

MARY C. KIMMEL, MD
Assistant Professor, Department of Psychiatry, Medical Director, Perinatal Psychiatry Inpatient Unit, The University of North Carolina at Chapel Hill, Chapel Hill, North Carolina

HRISTINA KOLEVA, MD
Clinical Associate Professor, Department of Psychiatry, University of Iowa, Iowa City, Iowa

SAMANTHA MELTZER-BRODY, MD, MPH
Associate Professor, Department of Psychiatry, Director, Perinatal Psychiatry Program, UNC Center for Women's Mood Disorders, The University of North Carolina at Chapel Hill, Chapel Hill, North Carolina

LAUREN M. OSBORNE, MD
Assistant Professor of Psychiatry and Behavioral Sciences and Gynecology and Obstetrics, Women's Mood Disorders Center, Johns Hopkins School of Medicine, Baltimore, Maryland

NAFISA REZA, MD
Resident, Department of Psychiatry, Zucker Hillside Hospital, Northwell Health, Glen Oaks, New York

ALYSSA A. RHEINGOLD, PhD
Director of Clinical Operations, Professor, Department of Psychiatry and Behavioral Sciences, Medical University of South Carolina, National Crime Victims Research and Treatment Center (NCVRTC), Charleston, South Carolina

CRYSTAL SCHILLER, PhD
Assistant Professor, Department of Psychiatry, The University of North Carolina at Chapel Hill, Chapel Hill, North Carolina

JAMIE STANHISER, MD
Clinical Instructor, Reproductive Endocrinology and Infertility, The University of North Carolina at Chapel Hill, Chapel Hill, North Carolina

ANNE Z. STEINER, MD, MPH
Professor, Division Chief of Reproductive Endocrinology and Infertility, Duke University, Durham, North Carolina

THOMAS W. UHDE, MD
Professor and Chair, Department of Psychiatry and Behavioral Sciences, Medical University of South Carolina, Charleston, South Carolina

ALLISON K. WILKERSON, PhD
Assistant Professor, Department of Psychiatry and Behavioral Sciences, Medical University of South Carolina, Charleston, South Carolina

KATHERINE E. WILLIAMS, MD
Clinical Professor, Department of Psychiatry and Behavioral Sciences, Stanford University School of Medicine, Stanford, California

KATHERINE L. WISNER, MD, MS
Norman and Helen Asher Professor of Psychiatry and Behavioral Sciences and Obstetrics and Gynecology, Northwestern University Feinberg School of Medicine, Chicago, Illinois

Contents

> Bipolar disorder affects women throughout their childbearing years.
> During the perinatal period, women with bipolar disorder are vulnerable
> to depressive episode recurrences and have an increased risk for post-
> partum psychosis. Perinatal screening is critical to identify women at
> risk. Although medications are the mainstay of treatment, the choice
> of pharmacotherapy must be made by the patient based on a
> risk-benefit discussion with her physician. For optimal dosing in preg-
> nancy, therapeutic drug monitoring may be required to maintain effec-
> tive drug concentrations. Residual symptoms of bipolar depression
> are treatable with bright light therapy as an alternative to medication
> augmentation.

> This article provides information about medications used to treat peri-
> natal depression, including guidance around when to use certain med-
> ications and when to consult a mental health provider. For each group
> of medications, including selective serotonin reuptake inhibitors, seroto-
> nin norepinephrine reuptake inhibitors, mirtazapine, bupropion, lithium,
> atypical antipsychotics, and lamotrigine, the risks and benefits of
> treatment during pregnancy and lactation are reviewed, and unique
> qualities of each medication. A treatment algorithm is included, as
> well as a description of the Food and Drug Administration's approach
> to providing information about medications. The article also discusses
> hormone therapies and future directions for new pharmacologic
> treatments.

> This article provides a focused review of the evidence for several comple-
> mentary health approaches (ie, omega-3 fatty acids, folate, vitamin D,

Attention deficit hyperactivity disorder (ADHD) is a common neurobehavioral disorder affecting 3.2% of women. More women are taking psychostimulant medications, including during pregnancy. Although stimulant use does not appear to be associated with congenital malformations, there are inconsistent data about other obstetric risks, and no long-term neurodevelopmental data exist to inform clinical management decisions. This article summarizes the available data regarding perinatal exposure to psychostimulants. It also highlights the importance of the risk-risk analysis for clinicians and patients to consider, weighing risks of medication exposure to risks of ADHD during pregnancy, including driving safety and major impairment in occupational roles.

Opioid agonist therapy is the standard of care for pregnant women with opioid use disorder, but medication-assisted withdrawal from opioid agonist therapy is increasingly prevalent. The authors review the available literature evaluating the risks and benefits of medication-assisted withdrawal. They highlight the importance of supporting women in making an informed treatment choice that is best for them. Although it is tempting to choose medication-assisted withdrawal to decrease the risk of newborn opioid withdrawal, the authors caution against this practice. Facilitating treatment that assists pregnant women in recovery ultimately produces the best outcome for women and their children.

This article discusses the prevalence and timing of perinatal loss. The impact that perinatal grief has on psychological functioning is presented, including common grief reactions and the risk factors for complicated grief. The ways that perinatal grief is processed by each parent and the impact that it has on the relationships are also discussed. The role of the health care professional is outlined, and the process for them to assist grieving parents is outlined in 5 steps. The screening process and treatment of grieving parents are also presented.

This article reviews the prevalence and outcomes of perinatal intimate partner violence (IPV). Reported rates of perinatal IPV range from 3.7% to 9.0%. Perinatal IPV is associated with a multitude of mental and obstetric health outcomes that affect the mother and child. Perinatal medical providers have an opportunity to detect victims of IPV and facilitate services for this population. Screening, safety planning, and referral procedures are essential for addressing this public health problem.

Health care providers (HCPs) are often poorly prepared to respond to childhood sexual abuse (CSA) survivors' needs in reproductive health care. With few protocols addressing the CSA survivor population, HCPs struggle with delivering interventions that meet professional standards of care within the systemic constraints of reproductive health care. To bridge the gap that exists when the unwelcome guest of CSA enters the reproductive health care arena, it is important to understand the psychological influences of trauma that affect CSA survivors, the symptoms or behavioral cues that are commonly revealed, and therapeutic approaches that can facilitate positive patient-provider experiences in health care.

Psychosocial aspects of fertility, infertility, and assisted reproductive technology (ART) can significantly affect patients' sense of self-identity and personal agency, mental well-being, sexual and marital relationships, reproductive efficiency, compliance with treatment, and pregnancy outcomes. Research is needed to understand how stress, anxiety, depression, mood disorders, and psychotropic medications affect fertility and infertility treatment. The psychosocial implications of ART on our society include a shift toward older maternal age at conception, the complexities of third-party reproduction, and consideration for the psychological and socioeconomic barriers to receiving care. Clinicians must understand, screen for, and identify couples struggling with the psychological and social aspects of fertility and ART.

OBSTETRICS AND GYNECOLOGY CLINICS

ISSUE OF RELATED INTEREST

Psychiatric Clinics of North America, June 2017 (Vol. 40, No. 2)
Women's Mental Health
Susan G. Kornstein and Anita H. Clayton, *Editors*
Available at: http://www.psych.theclinics.com/

THE CLINICS ARE AVAILABLE ONLINE!
Access your subscription at:
www.theclinics.com

Foreword

Pregnancy: An Opportune Time to Evaluate and Treat Mental Health Disorders

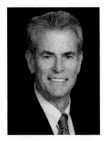

William F. Rayburn, MD, MBA
Consulting Editor

This issue of the *Obstetrics and Gynecology Clinics of North America* is dedicated to a contemporary and comprehensive look at perinatal mental health. The issue is capably edited by two well-recognized academicians in separate fields: a perinatal psychiatrist and maternal-fetal medicine specialist, Dr Constance Guille and Dr Roger Newman, respectively. I am now seeing more psychiatrists pursing expertise in women's behavioral health, especially in obstetrics, which is critical due to the insufficient number of experienced providers being available.

Pregnancy and the puerperium are at times sufficiently stressful to invoke or aggravate mental illness. Such illness may represent a recurrence or exacerbation of a presenting psychiatric disorder or may signal the onset of a new condition. In general, psychiatric disorders during pregnancy have been associated with less prenatal care, more substance abuse, and more peripartum psychiatric illness. Some, but not all, link maternal psychiatric illness with untoward outcomes, such as preterm birth, low birth weight, and perinatal mortality. It is a problem not only for the mother and newborn but also for the family and community. Pregnancy is an opportune time to provide individualized risk discussions, comparing the hazards of untreated mental illness with the known or unknown risks associated with treatment options.

Unfortunately, many mental health disorders, such as depression and anxiety, are not identified easily due to the stressors of pregnancy, thereby limiting access for affected women to emotional support and professional evaluation. Screening for mental illness is generally done at the first prenatal visit. Risk factors should include a personal or family history of mental illness; sexual, physical, or verbal abuse; substance abuse; and personality disorders. Repeat inquiry about these conditions should

Obstet Gynecol Clin N Am 45 (2018) xiii–xiv
https://doi.org/10.1016/j.ogc.2018.06.002
0889-8545/18/© 2018 Published by Elsevier Inc.

obgyn.theclinics.com

also be undertaken as gestation advances, after delivery, and during the initial post-partum visit.

The identification and treatment of common anxiety disorders, depression, bipolar disorder, and opioid use disorder are aptly covered in this issue. Well described are other important topics, such as perinatal intimate partner violence, management of attention and hyperactivity disorders, childhood sexual abuse survivors, and psychological functioning after pregnancy loss. Updates regarding perinatal sleep problems and psychosocial aspects of fertility and assisted reproductive technology are informative and timely.

This issue reviews principles of antenatal, intrapartum, and postpartum care of women with major mental disorders. Our patients deserve involvement in balanced and informed treatment decision making. Many psychotropic medications may be prescribed during pregnancy for the myriad of mental disorders. Some known and possible fetal and neonatal effects of treatment are described in each article, for example, studies implicating SSRIs with an increased teratogenic risk for fetal cardiac defects (paroxetine) and persistent pulmonary hypertension of the newborn. Although some psychotropic medications pass into breast milk, drug and metabolite levels are either very low or undetectable in most cases.

Evidence-based descriptions of information in this issue should prove to be helpful to both obstetrics and mental health providers. I appreciate the team effort of Dr Guille and Dr Newman in preparing this quality clinical reference that should have wide-spread appeal. The authors and coauthors form an expert group with much experience to share. A subsequent issue should prove to be helpful once additional clinical experience with outcomes are further clarified.

William F. Rayburn, MD, MBA
Department of Obstetrics and Gynecology
Continuing Medical Education and
Continuing Professional Development
University of New Mexico School of Medicine
MSC 10 5580, 1 University of New Mexico
Albuquerque, NM 87131-0001, USA

E-mail address:
WRayburn@salud.unm.edu

Preface

Treatment of Peripartum Mental Health Disorders: An Essential Element of Prenatal Care

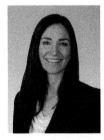
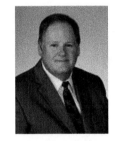

Constance Guille, MD, MSCR   Roger B. Newman, MD
Editors

Obstetricians and Gynecologists are acutely aware of the prevalence of maternal mental health disorders and the impact they can have on maternal, fetal, and newborn health and child development. Sadly, fewer than half of pregnant women with a mental health illness are identified in clinical settings. Among women who are identified, only 15% receive mental health treatment, fewer than 10% receive adequate treatment, and less than 5% achieve remission from their illness.

The shortfall in the recognition and treatment of peripartum mental health disorders is multifactorial. Obstetricians and Gynecologists are not typically provided with the necessary training to easily identify and adequately treat psychiatric disorders. Even when mental health problems are identified, mental health providers capable of or available to care for these women are frequently insufficient. The wait times for psychiatric appointments are often too long to be of use during pregnancy. Furthermore, women often refuse to seek mental health care in psychiatric settings, and significant barriers to accessing psychiatric care exist, such as stigma, fear of child welfare consequences, cost, inconvenience, and lack of adequate child care. Consequently, Obstetricians and Gynecologists are often faced with treating maternal psychiatric disorders in peripartum women: a fact that your clinical schedule reinforces virtually every day.

The goal of this issue is to provide Obstetricians and Gynecologists with practical clinical guidance for evidence-based pharmacologic and nonpharmacologic treatment options for common peripartum mental health problems, such as mood disorders, including Bipolar Disorder and Major Depression. In addition, we address the myriad of Anxiety Disorders and sleep disturbances that commonly present in pregnancy and provide guidance on treatments that are best suited for specific presentations.

Obstet Gynecol Clin N Am 45 (2018) xv–xvi
https://doi.org/10.1016/j.ogc.2018.06.001
0889-8545/18/© 2018 Published by Elsevier Inc.

Given the increasing prevalence of stimulant use among reproductive age women, we also include an article on the management of peripartum Attention Deficit/Hyperactivity Disorder. As you also well know, the national epidemic of increasing opioid misuse and abuse and overdose deaths in our country is mirrored in pregnancy. Our care of these women would be benefited by practical clinical guidance to manage this complex and growing high-risk population. A common theme throughout these articles is the need for patient-centered, individualized risk discussion inclusive of the hazards associated with untreated mental illness and the known and unknown risks associated with available treatment options, allowing women to make balanced and informed treatment decisions.

Other common peripartum mental health topics addressed within this issue include pregnancy loss, domestic violence, and previous sexual assault: all of which have a significant and negative short- and long-term impact on women's health and perinatal outcomes if not appropriately addressed with psychological care. While postpartum psychosis is an uncommon complication among peripartum women, we felt it was important to address the management of this illness since it is a true psychiatric emergency. Prompt and effective treatment is critical to maternal and newborn safety. Last, with the advancement and prevalence of assisted reproductive technology comes a unique set of medical decisions that can have profound psychological impact on women and their families. Thus, we dedicated an article to addressing this contemporary, evolving, and important topic.

Recognition and adequate treatment of maternal mental health disorders is a public health priority due to its significant impact on both short- and long-term women's health and child development. The provision of mental health care as an essential element of prenatal care is critical to the overall improvement of women's health. We are proud of our assembled authors and wish to thank them for their remarkable contributions. Without them, this symposium would not be the contemporary, comprehensive, and quality clinical reference on maternal mental health treatment that we believe it to be.

Constance Guille, MD, MSCR
Women's Reproductive Behavioral
Health Program
Department of Psychiatry and
Behavioral Sciences
Department of Obstetrics and Gynecology
Medical University of South Carolina
Institute of Psychiatry
67 President Street, MSC 861
Charleston, SC 29425, USA

Roger B. Newman, MD
Department of Obstetrics and Gynecology
Medical University of South Carolina
Clinical Science Building
96 Jonathan Lucas Street
Charleston, SC 29425, USA

E-mail addresses:
guille@musc.edu (C. Guille)
newmanr@musc.edu (R.B. Newman)

Treatment of Peripartum Bipolar Disorder

Crystal T. Clark, MD, MSc*, Katherine L. Wisner, MD, MS

KEYWORDS

- Bipolar disorder • Pregnancy • Lithium • Lamotrigine • Carbamazepine
- Antipsychotics • Light therapy • MDQ

KEY POINTS

- Women with bipolar disorder are vulnerable to episode recurrence during pregnancy and they have an increased risk for postpartum depression and psychosis.
- Pharmacotherapy is the mainstay of treatment for bipolar disorder and the benefits of medication management during pregnancy and lactation often justify the risks.
- Monthly therapeutic drug monitoring with dose adjustment is recommended for patients taking lithium and lamotrigine during pregnancy.
- Bright light therapy is an effective adjunct to treat bipolar depression.

INTRODUCTION

Bipolar disorder (BD) is characterized by chronic remitting and relapsing episodes of depression, hypomania, and mania. The lifetime prevalence is 4.4% (including all subtypes) of the United States population.[1] Men and women have a similar incidence of BD, but women are more likely to have depressive episodes, precipitous changes between depression and hypomania/mania (ie, rapid cycling), and episodes of both depressive and manic symptoms (ie, mixed states).[2] With an average age of onset at 18 years, women are affected throughout their reproductive years and pregnancy is a vulnerable time for episode recurrence. The mainstay of treatment for BD is pharmacotherapy and the goal is prevention of symptoms of BD during pregnancy and postpartum.

Compared with women with major depressive disorder, those with BD are at a greater risk for mood worsening immediately postpartum and are 50% more likely than those with major depression to have postpartum depression.[3] Women with BD are seven times more likely to be hospitalized for a first-time mood episode early

Disclosure Statement: The authors have no conflicts to disclose.
Department of Psychiatry and Behavioral Sciences, Northwestern University Feinberg School of Medicine, 676 St. Clair Street, Chicago, IL 60611, USA
* Corresponding author.
E-mail address: crystal.clark@northwestern.edu

postpartum.[4] Mental illness in the perinatal period increases the risk for suicide, a leading cause of maternal death.[5,6] With a 25% to 50% increased risk for psychosis—a 100-fold increase over the rate in the general population—women with BD are particularly vulnerable to severe postpartum mood worsening.[3] Clinicians must be able to distinguish between unipolar and bipolar depressive episodes to provide appropriate clinical management.

Optimizing pregnancy and postpartum outcomes for women with BD requires early identification, symptom monitoring, and effective treatment. This review focuses on the risk of untreated perinatal BD and treatment options. We discuss:

1. Screening for perinatal BD,
2. The risks of illness exposure,
3. The risks of pharmacotherapy during pregnancy and breastfeeding,
4. Effective dosing across childbearing, and
5. Nondrug treatments including bright light therapy and electroconvulsive therapy.

PATIENT EVALUATION OVERVIEW

Although manic and hypomanic episodes are diagnostic of BD, most episodes in the perinatal period are depressive. Acute episodes of bipolar and unipolar depression are clinically indistinguishable. The differentiation is based on the occurrence of previous manic or hypomanic episodes, which define bipolar 1 and bipolar 2 disorder, respectively. The distinction is important in the postpartum period, which confers a high risk for both recurrent and new onset BD. Manic and hypomanic episodes are distinguished by an elevated or irritable mood and increased energy that is present most of every day for four (hypomania) or seven (mania) consecutive days.[6] Patients must also have at least three or four (if an irritable mood is present) additional symptoms present including grandiosity, sleeping less than usual or not at all, rapid and verbose speech, racing thoughts, difficulty focusing, impulsive behavior, and/or increased goal directed activity at home or at work.[6] The onset of mood symptoms and the change in energy must not be attributable to the use of a substance or a medical comorbidity to meet criterion for BD. A personal history of postpartum depression, postpartum psychosis, or a family history of a first-degree relative with BD increases the risk for illness onset during the perinatal period. Ideally, during a preconception appointment, clinicians will inquire about diagnoses of mental illness, treatment with psychotropic medications, and/or family psychiatric history to guide the discussion of pregnancy management.

The US Preventive Services Task Force recommends depression screening for pregnant and postpartum women, but it does not mention strategies to differentiate unipolar from bipolar depression.[7] In a study by Wisner and colleagues[8] of 10,000 postpartum women in an urban obstetric setting, 22.6% of women with a positive depression screen (score of ≥ 10 on the Edinburgh Postnatal Depression Scale [EPDS]) were diagnosed with BD with a research diagnostic examination. None of the commonly used depression screens, such as the EPDS[9] (a 10-item, self-report scale, translated into 36 languages) and Patient Health Questionnaire (PHQ-9[10]; a 9-item, self-report instrument that has been validated in perinatal clinics) distinguish bipolar from unipolar depression.

The Mood Disorder Questionnaire (MDQ)[11] is a brief self-report screen for BD that takes approximately 5 minutes to complete. The MDQ includes 13 symptoms, the timing of symptoms, and the degree of impairment. A positive screen includes endorsement of seven symptoms occurring at the same time with moderate or serious impairment. Similar to the findings of Wisner and colleagues,[8] Merrill and colleagues[12] reported that 21.4% of perinatal women in an obstetric clinic screened with the EPDS screened positive for BD on the MDQ. In a study of postpartum women with a positive EPDS score (a score of $\geq$10), Clark and colleagues[13] found that the MDQ accurately identified 50% of women with BD according to a structured diagnostic interview. The identification rate was increased to 68% by excluding the impairment criterion. We recommend using the following MDQ screen criteria for perinatal women: (1) the presence of 7 symptoms and (2) endorsement that symptoms occurred at the same time. We advise screening with both the EPDS or PHQ-9 and the MDQ before treatment is initiated. Screening patients with the MDQ at the initial presentation during pregnancy and again at the first follow-up visit with an obstetrician increases detection of patients with BD. Although the MDQ includes questions about a history of manic symptoms, it is also a useful way to determine the presence of current symptoms.

Psychiatric evaluation is the next step for patients who screen positive on the MDQ. When psychiatric services are unavailable or will be delayed, obstetricians are in the best position to initiate treatment. A review of current or past effective medication regimens informs the treatment plan. Patients who are effectively treated may elect to continue their medication regimen to prevent episode recurrence. Continuation of pharmacotherapy will be most critical for patients who endorse rapid decompensation when medications are discontinued, hospitalizations for BD episodes, suicide attempts, psychotic episodes, poor response to medication trials, and/or long recovery times when resuming effective treatment regimens. For positive screens without a prior diagnosis, the MDQ is a useful tool to educate patients about BD symptoms.

After birth, women who have a diagnosis of BD or screen positive on the MDQ and who cannot access psychiatric care can be supported through follow-up with their obstetrician for symptom monitoring with the EPDS/PHQ-9 and MDQ as well as medication management. The function of monitoring is to assess for the onset or worsening of symptoms given the risk of postpartum psychosis, a psychiatric emergency, among women with BD (refer to Lauren M. Osborne's article, "Recognizing and Managing Postpartum Psychosis: A Clinical Guide for Obstetric Providers," in this issue).

PHARMACOLOGIC TREATMENT OPTIONS DURING PREGNANCY AND LACTATION

The choice to continue medication during pregnancy balances the risks of an untreated illness with the risks of medication exposure (**Fig. 1**). Untreated or undertreated BD during pregnancy is associated with poor birth outcomes independent of pharmacotherapy exposure, including preterm birth, low birth-weight, intrauterine growth retardation, small for gestational age, fetal distress, and adverse neurodevelopmental outcomes.[14] Women with untreated BD also have behavioral risk factors such as decreased compliance with prenatal care, poor nutrition, and high-risk behaviors (eg, sexual indiscretions and substance abuse) that jeopardize the fetus.[15] Impaired capacity to function may result in loss of employment, health care benefits, and social support. The biological and psychosocial risks of a BD episode are the justification for the risk of medication exposure.

Lithium, anticonvulsants (lamotrigine [LTG] and carbamazepine), and second-generation antipsychotics (aripiprazole, asenapine, lurasidone, olanzapine, immediate-release and extended-release quetiapine, risperidone, and ziprasidone) have Food and Drug Administration indications for the treatment of BD. Lithium and anticonvulsants are long-term maintenance treatments to prevent manic and

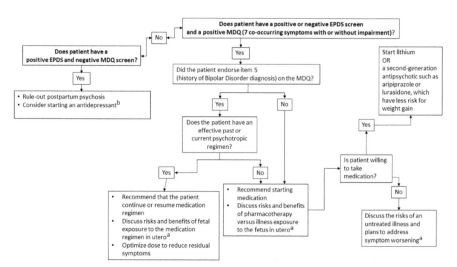

Fig. 1. Treatment algorithm. [a] Additional risk–benefit information and patient Fact Sheets available at Mother to Baby (mothertobaby.org). [b] Patients with a family history of bipolar disorder (item 4 of the Mood Disorder Questionnaire [MDQ]) require monitoring for antidepressant induced activation. EPDS, Edinburgh Postnatal Depression Scale.

depressive episodes. Similarly, second-generation antipsychotics are prescribed for maintenance treatment and are also effective treatments for acute mania. Although the anticonvulsant valproic acid is an effective mood stabilizer, other drugs are preferred for women of childbearing age owing to the risk for birth defects and neurodevelopmental delays. Carbamazepine is typically continued for patients for whom another option would not be as effective or when the patient presents pregnant and the risk of changing to another drug with unknown efficacy increases the risk for poor outcomes owing to recurrence.

Abrupt discontinuation of psychotropic medications is associated with an increased risk for illness recurrence. Women with BD who discontinue their medications before or during pregnancy have a 71% risk of recurrence with new episodes occurring most frequently in the first trimester.[16] Recurrent illness during pregnancy is associated with a 66% increase in the risk of postpartum episodes.[16] Women who only have a history of postpartum psychosis are less likely to have a recurrence of BD during pregnancy.[17] For these women, medication may be tapered and discontinued during pregnancy and resumed immediately postpartum to prevent postpartum psychosis.[17]

There are physiologic changes during pregnancy that result in decreases in the plasma concentrations of many psychotropic medications. Therapeutic drug monitoring is essential for lithium and LTG therapy during the perinatal period. Serial assessment of symptoms across pregnancy is also critical to make dose adjustments. Because depressive episodes are the most common mood recurrences during the perinatal period, assessment with the EPDS or the PHQ-9 is advised at each office visit. Although antidepressants are often used as adjunctive treatment, monotherapy risks mania induction and destabilization for women with bipolar 1 disorder. We summarize treatment recommendations, including symptom and therapeutic dose monitoring, as well as dose adjustments across childbearing for commonly prescribed medications.

Mood Stabilizers

Lithium
Congenital malformations Fetal exposure to lithium has been associated with an increased risk for cardiac abnormalities. The risk for Ebstein's anomaly with first trimester exposure is 1 (0.1%) to 2 in 1000 (0.2%), but the absolute risk remains low.[18] Folate supplementation with 5 mg reduces the risk and severity of congenital heart disease by suppressing lithium-induced potentiation of a signaling pathway that inhibits genes important to initiating cardiogenesis.[19] No other congenital malformations have been associated with lithium exposure.

Infant outcomes Adverse outcomes of in utero lithium exposure are associated with increased risk for diabetes insipidus, respiratory problems, tachycardia, transient neonatal hypothyroidism, tremor, and neuromuscular complications.[20–22] The incidences of these outcomes have not been defined and are based on a few case reports. Elevated maternal plasma and umbilical cord lithium concentrations at delivery increase the risk for adverse neonatal outcomes including neuromuscular, central nervous system, and respiratory complications.[23] Children exposed to lithium in utero have not been reported to experience neurodevelopmental delays.[24]

Management during pregnancy and postpartum Strategies to minimize fetal exposure and maintain efficacy include using the lowest effective dose, prescribing lithium twice daily to avoid high peak serum concentrations, and regular monitoring of lithium serum concentrations.[25] Lithium has a narrow therapeutic window (0.6–1.0 mEq/L) and serum concentrations are obtained at 12 hours after dosing for therapeutic dose monitoring.[26] Lithium is exclusively eliminated by the kidney; as a result, lithium serum concentrations begin decreasing during the first trimester of pregnancy owing to increases in the glomerular filtration rate.[27,28] The lithium dose must be increased to maintain effective concentrations. Because the therapeutic lithium concentration varies greatly among women, the effective serum concentration is established before pregnancy. If a therapeutic concentration has not been established, the lithium dose is titrated to a concentration within the therapeutic range. Throughout pregnancy, lithium concentrations are monitored monthly with dose adjustment as appropriate.[25] For women with first trimester exposure, fetal echocardiography and a level 2 ultrasound examination is recommended at 16 to 18 weeks of gestation to evaluate for anomalies.[20,25] Holding the lithium dose at the onset of labor or 24 to 48 hours before a planned labor induction or cesarean section prevents adverse outcomes associated with high lithium concentrations at delivery.[23] After delivery, the lithium dose is immediately adjusted back to the prepregnancy therapeutic dose. If lithium was initiated during pregnancy, lithium levels are checked at the end of the first postpartum week and repeated weekly to achieve a concentration in the therapeutic range and prevent toxicity.

Breastfeeding Few cases of adverse effects have been reported for newborns exposed to lithium exclusively through breast milk. Published cases have included newborns who had cyanosis, elevated thyroid-stimulating hormone, and lithium toxicity who were also exposed to lithium in utero.[29,30] In all cases, the adverse effects were associated with maternal toxicity or compromised health status of the infant (ie, infection, prematurity).

Data from case series estimate that newborns exposed to lithium through breast milk have serum lithium concentrations that are one-fourth of the maternal serum lithium concentration.[31] LACTMED advises that women who have full-term infants can take lithium and breastfeed with monitoring for infant restlessness or difficulty feeding.[32] Lithium exposure in infants with an infection, dehydration, or premature birth increases the risk of adverse effects and fluid supplementation and pumping, instead of breastfeeding, is appropriate until the infant is evaluated and lithium toxicity is ruled out. Maternal and infant lithium levels are obtained for an infant with changes in behavior, increased sedation, signs of dehydration, restlessness, and difficulty feeding.[33] Laboratory monitoring of infant lithium serum concentrations, thyroid-stimulating hormone, blood urea nitrogen, and creatinine are only advised for clinical concerns.

Lamotrigine
Congenital malformation LTG exposure has not been associated with an increased risk of congenital malformations. Four epilepsy registries reported the rate of major congenital malformation (MCM) to be between 2.0% and 2.9% for a combined total of 6498 pregnant women with first trimester exposure to LTG, which is similar to the 3% to 5% MCM rate in the general population.[34–37] The European Registry of Antiepileptic Drugs and Pregnancy[35] and the United Kingdom Epilepsy and Pregnancy Register[38] previously reported a dose-related increase in MCMs for LTG doses greater than 200 mg and of greater than 300 mg/d, respectively but a recent analysis from a larger sample did not replicate a significant difference in the rate of MCMs for low-dose (</= to 200 mg) versus high-dose (> 400 mg) LTG.[37] A 6-fold increased risk for cleft palate was reported from the North American Pregnancy AED Registry in 2008,[39] but this finding has not been reproducible. A recent (2016) population-based case-control study did not observe an increase in orofacial cleft or cleft palate compared with babies not exposed to LTG.[40] Given the favorable reproductive profile of LTG, it is a preferred option among patients and physicians.

Infant outcomes Pregnancy complications such as preterm birth, miscarriages, and stillbirths have not been associated with in utero LTG exposure.[41] Studies suggest that IQ scores are average or potentially above average in children with in utero exposure to LTG and there are no significant adverse effects.[42,43]

Management during pregnancy and postpartum During pregnancy, LTG clearance increases by as much as 330%.[44] The accelerated metabolism is attributed to the increasing concentrations of estradiol across pregnancy and the associated upregulation of the primary metabolic enzyme for LTG, uridine diphosphate-glucuronosyl transferase (UGT1A4). Decreasing LTG concentrations across pregnancy owing to increased clearance requires dose adjustments to maintain therapeutic LTG concentrations. In nonpregnant patients, the recommended maintenance dose of LTG for BD is 200 mg, but effective doses range from 100 to 500 mg.[45,46] During pregnancy, patients may require double to triple their prepregnancy dose. Because a therapeutic range for LTG has not been determined for the treatment of BD and is variable among individuals, a woman's effective concentration is determined by checking her trough LTG serum concentration (ie, the lowest serum concentration of a drug, which is right before the next dose is scheduled) before pregnancy.[47]

　　LTG concentrations begin decreasing as early as 10 weeks of gestation and plateau in the third trimester. Monthly monitoring of trough concentrations is necessary to make timely dose adjustments.[47] If more convenient for the patient, blood draws may be obtained at a consistent time of day, instead of at trough, for comparability between timepoints. Patients are also advised to take LTG twice a day and at the same time each day to maintain stable concentrations.

If the LTG dose is increased during pregnancy, an immediate taper to the prepregnancy dose within 2 weeks postpartum is critical owing to the rapid decline in LTG clearance postpartum. Based on an adaptation of neurology clinical guidelines[48,49] we recommend an immediate postbirth decrease in dose by 25% to prevent toxicity symptoms of ataxia, dizziness and double or blurred vision as well as prevent the transfer of high concentrations of LTG through breastfeeding. The dose must be further decreased every 3 to 4 days until the prepregnancy dose is reached.[49]

Breastfeeding Maternal-to-infant transfer of LTG in breast milk has been reported in 40 cases and plasma concentrations in infants are 6% to 50% of the maternal plasma concentration.[47] Although infants do not have the full capacity to metabolize LTG by glucuronidation until 6 months of age,[50] there are no known contraindications to breastfeeding in full-term, healthy neonates.[51] There have been no reports of rashes associated with breast milk exposure to LTG. Only 1 case reported by Nordmo and colleagues[52] (2009) of an adverse effect associated with breast milk exposure to LTG has been published. The mother had toxic levels of LTG and exposed her infant through breast milk. This report underscores the importance of dose adjustments back to the prepregnancy baseline dose postpartum. If a woman taking LTG breastfeeds and her infant has difficulty feeding or is lethargic, obtaining an evaluation of the infant by a pediatrician as well as a maternal and infant LTG serum concentration rules out toxicity. Neurodevelopment at 6 years of age for children exposed to LTG through breast milk after exposure in utero is not significantly different from children without breast milk exposure to LTG after exposure in utero. Infants who were breastfed had higher IQ scores on average.[53]

Carbamazepine
Congenital malformation Carbamazepine therapy during pregnancy is associated with an increase in congenital malformations. In a metaanalysis of 21 prospective studies and 1255 exposures to carbamazepine in utero, 6.7% of infants had a major defect compared with 2.34% of controls.[54] In a majority of the studies, women had first trimester exposure. The most common malformations associated with carbamazepine monotherapy were neural tube, cardiac, and urinary tract defects. First trimester exposure, specifically, was linked to fingernail hypoplasia, developmental delays, and craniofacial malformations. Treatments combining carbamazepine with other anticonvulsants increased the risk for malformation and taking 2 additional antiepileptic drugs were linked to cardiac, cleft palate, and urinary tract abnormalities.[55] Oxcarbazepine is an anticonvulsant with off-label use commonly used for BD and is thought to have less teratogenic effects than carbamazepine, although more investigation is needed.

Infant outcomes Carbamazepine exposure in utero is linked to reduced fetal head growth.[54,56,57] Although carbamazepine is associated with restricted intrauterine growth, birth weight, and body length in some studies,[58] other investigations have not found these variables to differ significantly from controls.[56] Two reports of toxicity have been published including a case of transient hepatic toxicity and hyperbilirubinemia.[59]

Exposure to carbamazepine in utero has not been associated with an effect on IQ in prospective, retrospective, or registry-based studies.[60] A decrease in verbal ability compared with controls was found in a recent prospective study (2015) of children born to women with epilepsy and blindly assessed at 6 years of age after exposure to carbamazepine during gestation.[43] This finding contradicted a previous report that verbal IQ was not significantly different from controls in a similarly designed investigation.[61]

Management during pregnancy and postpartum During pregnancy, unbound and free carbamazepine serum levels do not significantly change and therapeutic drug monitoring is not clinically useful.[62] Because carbamazepine therapy is associated with vitamin K deficiency, experts recommend women take 20 mg/d of oral vitamin K during the last month of pregnancy.[25] Vitamin K should also be administered to the newborn, 1 mg intramuscularly.

Breastfeeding For women taking carbamazepine and breastfeeding, 32% to 80% of the maternal serum carbamazepine is found in the breast milk. Interindividual variability is wide because the active metabolite is poorly excreted in the breast milk. Breastfeeding is supported for women taking carbamazepine, but any concerns for adequate growth or lethargy are evaluated by the pediatrician, including checking of maternal and infant serum concentrations.[63,64]

Second-generation antipsychotics

Second-generation antipsychotics have Food and Drug Administration indications for the acute management of psychotic illnesses, acute mania, and maintenance treatment for BD. Additionally, they are combined with mood stabilizers for patients who have achieved a partial response despite dose optimization. With the increasing number of second-generation antipsychotics on the market, fewer first-generation antipsychotic medications (eg, haloperidol, perphenazine, fluphenazine) are prescribed. This trend is due to the occurrence of fewer extrapyramidal side effects and increased patient tolerability compared with first-generation antipsychotics. Although first-generation antipsychotics are effective and have more published data during pregnancy, we focus on second-generation antipsychotics because they are more commonly prescribed and have more than doubled in use during pregnancy in the United States.[65]

Congenital malformation Second-generation antipsychotics are not associated with an increased risk of MCMs when compared with healthy controls, with the exception of risperidone. An increased risk for cardiac malformation with a relative risk of 1.26 after adjustment for potential confounding variables has been reported for risperidone but more investigation is needed.[66] The national pregnancy registry data for second-generation antipsychotics from the Massachusetts General Hospital has had 303 women with second-generation antipsychotic exposure complete the study and the risk of major malformation was not found to be beyond that of the general population.[67] A recent investigation of 9258 women enrolled in Medicaid with a live-born infant and at least 1 filled prescription for a second-generation antipsychotic during pregnancy did not find an increased risk for congenital malformations.[66] Among women not exposed to a second-generation antipsychotic during pregnancy, 32.7 per 100 births had a congenital malformation compared with 44.5 per 1000 births among women who took a second-generation antipsychotic. The rate of malformation is consistent with the 3% to 5% rate in the general population. More infant developmental outcome data related to general second-generation antipsychotic use and individual second-generation antipsychotic medications are needed.

Infant outcomes Some investigators report an increased risk of low birth weight and small for gestational age in babies exposed to second-generation antipsychotics in utero.[68,69] In many studies, the effect of illness exposure on birth outcomes has not been determined. Lin and colleagues[68] (2010) noted that the risk for low birth weight, preterm birth, small for gestational age, and large for gestational age was similar in women with schizophrenia who were treated with a second-generation antipsychotic compared with untreated women with schizophrenia. An increased risk of obesity owing to second-generation antipsychotic-related weight gain and gestational diabetes has been reported as an independent risk factor of second-generation antipsychotic treatment and increases the risk of poor outcomes such as macrosomia, impaired growth, and preterm birth.[69–71] The weight-neutral properties of aripiprazole and lurasidone make them preferred second-generation antipsychotics during the perinatal period. Alternatively, olanzapine and quetiapine are associated with excessive weight gain, which may increase the risk for poor birth outcomes. Consistent with the recommendations from the American College of Obstetricians and Gynecologists for obesity management, monitoring body mass index beginning at the first prenatal visit and reinforcing weight management techniques of dietary control, exercise, and behavior modification are necessary to prevent excessive weight gain. High-risk obstetric care is recommended. Patient referrals to the National Registry at Massachusetts General Hospital are encouraged to obtain more data on pregnancy outcomes, which will help to inform reproductive risk.[72]

In a small study of infants, in utero second-generation antipsychotic exposure was associated with a delay in cognitive, motor, and social/emotional development at 2 months.[73] At 6 and 12 months of age, no delay was present. In a prospective study of controls versus infants exposed to a second-generation antipsychotic, no significant differences were found at 2 months of age for cognitive, motor, and social/emotional functioning or for language.[74]

Breastfeeding Olanzapine, risperidone, and quetiapine have the most available data to inform exposure risk during breastfeeding. These agents have milk/plasma ratios (the estimate of concentration in maternal serum to milk) that are less than 1, and relative infant dose ratios that are less than 10%, reflecting acceptable infant exposure.[75] Information on maternal serum-to-milk transfer is limited for other second-generation antipsychotics such as lurasidone and aripiprazole. Although prevalence has not been established, adverse events are infrequent, mild, and include somnolence, irritability, tremor, and insomnia as well as speech, motor, and mental delays.

Dose management during pregnancy and postpartum Doses of second-generation antipsychotics may need to be increased owing to the increased metabolism by the cytochrome P450 system including CYP2D6 and CYP3A4 enzymes.[76] During pregnancy, enzyme activity of CYP2D6 increases beginning early in the second trimester and increases further as the pregnancy progresses.[77] Risperidone is predominantly metabolized by CYP2D6 and may decrease in concentration across pregnancy, resulting in a need for a dose increase. Lurasidone, aripiprazole, and quetiapine concentrations may also decrease across gestation because they are substrates of CYP3A4, which is also induced in pregnancy.[77,78] Because a therapeutic concentration is not established for second-generation antipsychotics and laboratory tests to check serum concentrations are not standard, symptom assessment at each office visit informs the need for a dose adjustment. Worsening symptoms for patients who were previously taking a second-generation antipsychotic and without symptoms suggest a decline in the preconception serum concentration and requires a dose increase. Postpartum, doses must be decreased to the original preconception dose to prevent adverse side effects and toxicity.

NONPHARMACOLOGIC TREATMENT
Bright Light Therapy

Bright light therapy is an evidenced-based treatment for seasonal depression that consists of exposure to broad spectrum light. Although many women with BD are unable to use alternatives to pharmacotherapy as their only treatment, bright light therapy is an effective augmentation strategy for the treatment of residual bipolar depression symptoms in patients taking an antimanic agent. It has not been associated with any reproductive risks and is an acceptable treatment among pregnant women.[79] The mechanism for symptom reduction is unclear and is attributed to the stabilization of the circadian rhythm and to a modulating effect on neurotransmitters such as 5HT that impact depression. Like all antidepressant treatments, light therapy can precipitate mania in women. It is contraindicated for women in manic, hypomanic, or mixed (ie, both depressive and manic symptoms) mood states. Patients who report excessive irritability are often in a mixed episode and, in these instances, light therapy is avoided. Side effects of bright light therapy include headache, nausea, and jitteriness.

The evidence-based apparatus for light therapy is a fluorescent box with a broad spectrum, ultraviolet-blocked light that provides 10,000 lux and is available commercially. In a recent double-blinded randomized controlled trial, Sit and colleagues[80] found that adjunctive midday bright light therapy with 7000 lux remitted depressive symptoms in 68% of depressed nonpregnant adults with bipolar 1 and bipolar 2 disorder compared with 22% in the control group. None of the patients in the treatment group experienced an onset of manic symptoms. Per Sit and colleagues' findings, therapy is recommended as follows:

1. With concurrent use of an antimanic agent,
2. Midday (between 12:00 PM and 2:30 PM),
3. Starting with 15 minutes a day for week one and increasing by 15 minutes a day each week until 60 minutes is reached at week 4, and
4. For a duration of 6 weeks.

Women with bipolar depression sit 12 to 14 inches away from the box, which is situated at or above eye-level. Additional information can be found on the nonprofit Center for Environmental Therapeutics (www.CET.org).

TREATMENT RESISTANCE
Electroconvulsive Therapy

Electroconvulsive therapy is a longstanding, safe, and effective procedure of passing electric currents through the brain to reduce severe mental health symptoms. Electroconvulsive therapy is completed under general anesthesia and is an effective option for perinatal patients who have a severe mood episode and have not responded to medication, lack ability for self-care (ie, unable to get out of bed, eat, or drink), are suicidal, or are psychotic.[81] Prolonged debilitations may jeopardize the fetus or newborn owing to poor self-care and functional incapacity. We recommend that patients who have not responded to medication after 3 medication trials or are an imminent risk to themselves have a consultation with a psychiatrist and be considered for electroconvulsive therapy.

SUMMARY

The perinatal period is a vulnerable time for the onset or reemergence of BD symptoms, especially those of bipolar depression. Screening with the MDQ in addition

---

Box 1
Professional and patient mental health resources

OTIS – Mother To Baby (provides professional and patient consultation about medication exposure during pregnancy and while breastfeeding based on evidenced based information. "Fact Sheets" for patients available on the website)
- http://www.mothertobaby.org/
- Toll-Free: 1 to 866 to 626 to 6847

Postpartum Support
- PSI, Postpartum Support International - www.postpartum.net

Women's Mental Health Center at Massachusetts General Hospital (for pregnancy, postpartum, perimenopause, premenstrual dysphoric disorder information)
- https://womensmentalhealth.org/

National Pregnancy Registry for Atypical Antipsychotics Registry, Massachusetts General Hospital
- www.womensmentalhealth.org/pregnancyregistry
- Toll-Free:1 to 866 to 961 to 2388

Center for Environmental Therapeutics (bright light therapy)
- www.CET.org

---

to the EPDS or PHQ-9 depression screen is a critical step in differentiating unipolar depression from bipolar depression to establish an optimal treatment plan. Pharmacotherapy is the most effective treatment for most women with BD, and the risks and benefits of exposure to medication versus untreated illness during pregnancy must be considered for each woman. Women with BD who continue medication in pregnancy and postpartum reduce their risk for episode recurrence as well as the onset of postpartum depression and postpartum psychosis. If available and indicated, medication combined with bright light therapy optimizes treatment for women with bipolar depression. When psychiatric services are limited, use of professional and patient mental health resources as shown in **Box 1** are advised.

REFERENCES

1. Merikangas KR, Akiskal HS, Angst J, et al. Lifetime and 12-month prevalence of bipolar spectrum disorder in the National Comorbidity Survey replication. Arch Gen Psychiatry 2007;64(5):543–52.
2. Leibenluft E. Issues in the treatment of women with bipolar illness. J Clin Psychiatry 1997;58(Suppl 15):5–11.
3. Sit DK, Wisner KL. Identification of postpartum depression. Clin Obstet Gynecol 2009;52(3):456–68.
4. Terp IM, Mortensen PB. Post-partum psychoses. Clinical diagnoses and relative risk of admission after parturition. Br J Psychiatry 1998;172(6):521–6.
5. Cantwell R, Clutton-Brock T, Cooper G, et al. Saving mothers' lives: reviewing maternal deaths to make motherhood safer: 2006-2008. The eighth report of the confidential enquiries into maternal deaths in the United Kingdom. BJOG 2011;118(Suppl 1):1–203.
6. American Psychiatric Association. Diagnostic and statistical manual of mental disorders. 5th edition. Washington, DC: American Psychiatric Publishing; 2013.
7. O'Connor E, Rossom RC, Henninger M, et al. Primary care screening for and treatment of depression in pregnant and postpartum women: evidence report

and systematic review for the US Preventive Services Task Force. JAMA 2016; 315(4):388–406.

8. Wisner KL, Sit DK, McShea MC, et al. Onset timing, thoughts of self-harm, and diagnoses in postpartum women with screen-positive depression findings. JAMA Psychiatry 2013;70(5):490–8.

9. Cox JL, Holden JM, Sagovsky R. Detection of postnatal depression. Development of the 10-item Edinburgh Postnatal Depression Scale. Br J Psychiatry 1987;150:782–6.

10. Kroenke K, Spitzer RL, Williams JB. The PHQ-9: validity of a brief depression severity measure. J Gen Intern Med 2001;16(9):606–13.

11. Hirschfeld RM, Williams JB, Spitzer RL, et al. Development and validation of a screening instrument for bipolar spectrum disorder: the Mood Disorder Questionnaire. Am J Psychiatry 2000;157(11):1873–5.

12. Merrill L, Mittal L, Nicoloro J, et al. Screening for bipolar disorder during pregnancy. Arch Womens Ment Health 2015;18(4):579–83.

13. Clark CT, Sit DK, Driscoll K, et al. Does screening with the MDQ and EPDS improve identification of bipolar disorder in an obstetrical sample? Depress Anxiety 2015;32(7):518–26.

14. Jablensky AV, Morgan V, Zubrick SR, et al. Pregnancy, delivery, and neonatal complications in a population cohort of women with schizophrenia and major affective disorders. Am J Psychiatry 2005;162(1):79–91.

15. Leight KL, Fitelson EM, Weston CA, et al. Childbirth and mental disorders. Int Rev Psychiatry 2010;22(5):453–71.

16. Viguera AC, Whitfield T, Baldessarini RJ, et al. Risk of recurrence in women with bipolar disorder during pregnancy: prospective study of mood stabilizer discontinuation. Am J Psychiatry 2007;164(12):1817–24 [quiz: 1923].

17. Bergink V, Bouvy PF, Vervoort JS, et al. Prevention of postpartum psychosis and mania in women at high risk. Am J Psychiatry 2012;169(6):609–15.

18. Cohen LS, Friedman JM, Jefferson JW, et al. A reevaluation of risk of in utero exposure to lithium. JAMA 1994;271(2):146–50.

19. Huhta JC, Linask K. When should we prescribe high-dose folic acid to prevent congenital heart defects? Curr Opin Cardiol 2015;30(1):125–31.

20. Diav-Citrin O, Shechtman S, Tahover E, et al. Pregnancy outcome following in utero exposure to lithium: a prospective, comparative, observational study. Am J Psychiatry 2014;171(7):785–94.

21. Blake LD, Lucas DN, Aziz K, et al. Lithium toxicity and the parturient: case report and literature review. Int J Obstet Anesth 2008;17(2):164–9.

22. Kozma C. Neonatal toxicity and transient neurodevelopmental deficits following prenatal exposure to lithium: another clinical report and a review of the literature. Am J Med Genet A 2005;132A(4):441–4.

23. Newport DJ, Viguera AC, Beach AJ, et al. Lithium placental passage and obstetrical outcome: implications for clinical management during late pregnancy. Am J Psychiatry 2005;162(11):2162–70.

24. van der Lugt NM, van de Maat JS, van Kamp IL, et al. Fetal, neonatal and developmental outcomes of lithium-exposed pregnancies. Early Hum Dev 2012;88(6): 375–8.

25. Yonkers KA, Wisner KL, Stowe Z, et al. Management of bipolar disorder during pregnancy and the postpartum period. Am J Psychiatry 2004;161(4):608–20.

26. Deligiannidis KM, Byatt N, Freeman MP. Pharmacotherapy for mood disorders in pregnancy: a review of pharmacokinetic changes and clinical recommendations for therapeutic drug monitoring. J Clin Psychopharmacol 2014;34(2):244–55.

27. Schou M, Amdisen A, Steenstrup OR. Lithium and pregnancy. II. Hazards to women given lithium during pregnancy and delivery. Br Med J 1973;2(5859): 137–8.

28. Wesseloo R, Wierdsma AI, van Kamp IL, et al. Lithium dosing strategies during pregnancy and the postpartum period. Br J Psychiatry 2017;211(1):31–6.

29. Tunnessen WW Jr, Hertz CG. Toxic effects of lithium in newborn infants: a commentary. J Pediatr 1972;81(4):804–7.

30. Skausig OB, Schou M. Breast feeding during lithium therapy. Ugeskr laeger 1977;139(7):400–1 [in Danish].

31. Viguera AC, Newport DJ, Ritchie J, et al. Lithium in breast milk and nursing infants: clinical implications. Am J Psychiatry 2007;164(2):342–5.

32. LactMed. Lithium. Available at: http://toxnet.nlm.nih.gov/cgi-bin/sis/search2/r? dbs+lactmed:@term+@DOCNO+293. Accessed June 18, 2018.

33. Bogen DL, Sit D, Genovese A, et al. Three cases of lithium exposure and exclusive breastfeeding. Arch Womens Ment Health 2012;15(1):69–72.

34. Hernandez-Diaz S, Smith CR, Shen A, et al. Comparative safety of antiepileptic drugs during pregnancy. Neurology 2012;78(21):1692–9.

35. Tomson T, Battino D, Bonizzoni E, et al. Dose-dependent risk of malformations with antiepileptic drugs: an analysis of data from the EURAP epilepsy and pregnancy registry. Lancet Neurol 2011;10(7):609–17.

36. Cunnington MC, Weil JG, Messenheimer JA, et al. Final results from 18 years of the International Lamotrigine Pregnancy Registry. Neurology 2011;76(21): 1817–23.

37. Campbell E, Kennedy F, Russell A, et al. Malformation risks of antiepileptic drug monotherapies in pregnancy: updated results from the UK and Ireland Epilepsy and Pregnancy Registers. J Neurol Neurosurg Psychiatry 2014;85(9):1029–34.

38. Morrow J, Russell A, Guthrie E, et al. Malformation risks of antiepileptic drugs in pregnancy: a prospective study from the UK Epilepsy and Pregnancy Register. J Neurol Neurosurg Psychiatry 2006;77:193–8.

39. Holmes LB, Baldwin EJ, Smith CR, et al. Increased frequency of isolated cleft palate in infants exposed to lamotrigine during pregnancy. Neurology 2008;70(22 Pt 2):2152–8.

40. Dolk H, Wang H, Loane M, et al. Lamotrigine use in pregnancy and risk of orofacial cleft and other congenital anomalies. Neurology 2016;86(18):1716–25.

41. Pariente G, Leibson T, Shulman T, et al. Pregnancy outcomes following in utero exposure to lamotrigine: a systematic review and meta-analysis. CNS Drugs 2017;31(6):439–50.

42. Rihtman T, Parush S, Ornoy A. Developmental outcomes at preschool age after fetal exposure to valproic acid and lamotrigine: cognitive, motor, sensory and behavioral function. Reprod Toxicol 2013;41:115–25.

43. Baker GA, Bromley RL, Briggs M, et al. IQ at 6 years after in utero exposure to antiepileptic drugs: a controlled cohort study. Neurology 2015;84(4):382–90.

44. Pennell PB, Newport DJ, Stowe ZN, et al. The impact of pregnancy and childbirth on the metabolism of lamotrigine. Neurology 2004;62(2):292–5.

45. GlaxoSmithKline. Lamictal Medication Guide. 2016.

46. Clabrese JR, Suppes T, Bowden CL, et al. A double-blind, placebo-controlled, prophylaxis study of lamotrigine in rapid-cycling bipolar disorder. J Clin Psychiatry 2000;61:841–50.

47. Clark CT, Klein AM, Perel JM, et al. Lamotrigine dosing for pregnant patients with bipolar disorder. Am J Psychiatry 2013;170(11):1240–7.

48. Sabers A. Algorithm for lamotrigine dose adjustment before, during, and after pregnancy. Acta Neurol Scand 2012;126(1):e1–4.

49. Pennell P, Peng L, Newport D, et al. Lamotrigine in pregnancy: clearance, therapeutic drug monitoring, and seizure frequency. Neurology 2008;70(22 Part 2): 2130–6.

50. Strassburg CP, Strassburg A, Kneip S, et al. Developmental aspects of human hepatic drug glucuronidation in young children and adults. Gut 2002;50(2): 259–65.

51. LactMed. Lamotrigine. Available at: http://toxnet.nlm.nih.gov/cgi-bin/sis/search2/r?dbs+lactmed:@term+@DOCNO+399. Accessed June 18, 2018.

52. Nordmo E, Aronsen L, Wasland K, et al. Severe apnea in an infant exposed to lamotrigine in breast milk. Ann Pharmacother 2009;43(11):1893–7.

53. Meador KJ, Baker GA, Browning N, et al. Breastfeeding in children of women taking antiepileptic drugs: cognitive outcomes at age 6 years. JAMA Pediatr 2014; 168(8):729–36.

54. Diav-Citrin O, Shechtman S, Arnon J, et al. Is carbamazepine teratogenic? A prospective controlled study of 210 pregnancies. Neurology 2001;57(2):321–4.

55. Matalon S, Schechtman S, Goldzweig G, et al. The teratogenic effect of carbamazepine: a meta-analysis of 1255 exposures. Reprod Toxicol 2002;16(1):9–17.

56. Wide K, Winbladh B, Tomson T, et al. Body dimensions of infants exposed to antiepileptic drugs in utero: observations spanning 25 years. Epilepsia 2000;41(7): 854–61.

57. Almgren M, Kallen B, Lavebratt C. Population-based study of antiepileptic drug exposure in utero–influence on head circumference in newborns. Seizure 2009; 18(10):672–5.

58. Bertollini R, Kallen B, Mastroiacovo P, et al. Anticonvulsant drugs in monotherapy. Effect on the fetus. Eur J Epidemiol 1987;3(2):164–71.

59. Frey B, Schubiger G, Musy JP. Transient cholestatic hepatitis in a neonate associated with carbamazepine exposure during pregnancy and breast-feeding. Eur J Pediatr 1990;150(2):136–8.

60. Haskey C, Galbally M. Mood stabilizers in pregnancy and child developmental outcomes: a systematic review. Aust N Z J Psychiatry 2017;51(11):1087–97.

61. Gaily E, Kantola-Sorsa E, Hiilesmaa V, et al. Normal intelligence in children with prenatal exposure to carbamazepine. Neurology 2004;62(1):28–32.

62. Johnson EL, Stowe ZN, Ritchie JC, et al. Carbamazepine clearance and seizure stability during pregnancy. Epilepsy Behav 2014;33:49–53.

63. Frey B, Braegger CP, Ghelfi D. Neonatal cholestatic hepatitis from carbamazepine exposure during pregnancy and breast feeding. Ann Pharmacother 2002; 36(4):644–7.

64. Ward RM, Bates BA, Benitz WE, et al. The transfer of drugs and other chemicals into human milk. Pediatrics 2001;108(3):776–89.

65. Toh S, Li Q, Cheetham TC, et al. Prevalence and trends in the use of antipsychotic medications during pregnancy in the U.S., 2001-2007: a population-based study of 585,615 deliveries. Arch Womens Ment Health 2013;16(2):149–57.

66. Huybrechts KF, Hernandez-Diaz S, Patorno E, et al. Antipsychotic use in pregnancy and the risk for congenital malformations. JAMA Psychiatry 2016;73(9): 938–46.

67. Cohen LS, Viguera AC, McInerney KA, et al. Reproductive safety of second-generation antipsychotics: current data from the massachusetts general hospital national pregnancy registry for atypical antipsychotics. Am J Psychiatry 2016; 173(3):263–70.

68. Lin HC, Chen IJ, Chen YH, et al. Maternal schizophrenia and pregnancy outcome: does the use of antipsychotics make a difference? Schizophr Res 2010;116(1):55–60.
69. Reis M, Källén B. Maternal use of antipsychotics in early pregnancy and delivery outcome. J Clin Psychopharmacol 2008;28(3):279–88.
70. Kessing LV, Thomsen AF, Mogensen UB, et al. Treatment with antipsychotics and the risk of diabetes in clinical practice. Br J Psychiatry 2010;197(4):266–71.
71. Hull HR, Dinger MK, Knehans AW, et al. Impact of maternal body mass index on neonate birthweight and body composition. Am J Obstet Gynecol 2008;198(4): 416.e1-6.
72. National Pregnant Registry for atypical antipshychotics 2016. Available at: https:// womensmentalhealth.org/clinical-and-research-programs/pregnancyregistry/ atypicalantipsychotic/. Accessed June 18, 2018.
73. Peng M, Gao K, Ding Y, et al. Effects of prenatal exposure to atypical antipsychotics on postnatal development and growth of infants: a case-controlled, prospective study. Psychopharmacology 2013;228(4):577–84.
74. Shao P, Ou J, Peng M, et al. Effects of clozapine and other atypical antipsychotics on infants development who were exposed to as fetus: a post-hoc analysis. PLoS One 2015;10(4):e0123373.
75. Uguz F. Second-generation antipsychotics during the lactation period: a comparative systematic review on infant safety. J Clin Psychopharmacol 2016;36(3): 244–52.
76. Ingelman-Sundberg M. Pharmacogenetics of cytochrome P450 and its applications in drug therapy: the past, present and future. Trends Pharmacol Sci 2004; 25(4):193–200.
77. Tracy TS, Venkataramanan R, Glover DD, et al. Temporal changes in drug metabolism (CYP1A2, CYP2D6 and CYP3A activity) during pregnancy. Am J obstetrics Gynecol 2005;192(2):633–9.
78. Hebert MF, Easterling T, Kirby B, et al. Effects of pregnancy on CYP3A and P-glycoprotein activities as measured by disposition of midazolam and digoxin: a University of Washington specialized center of research study. Clin Pharmacol Ther 2008;84(2):248–53.
79. Bais B, Kamperman AM, van der Zwaag MD, et al. Bright light therapy in pregnant women with major depressive disorder: study protocol for a randomized, double-blind, controlled clinical trial. BMC Psychiatry 2016;16(1):381.
80. Sit DK, McGowan J, Wiltrout C, et al. Adjunctive bright light therapy for bipolar depression: a randomized double-blind placebo-controlled trial. Am J Psychiatry 2017;175(2):131–9.
81. Haxton C, Kelly S, Young D, et al. The efficacy of electroconvulsive therapy in a perinatal population: a comparative pilot study. J ECT 2016;32(2):113–5.

Pharmacologic Treatment of Perinatal Depression

Mary C. Kimmel, MD*, Elizabeth Cox, MD, Crystal Schiller, PhD, Edith Gettes, MD, Samantha Meltzer-Brody, MD, MPH

KEYWORDS

- Depression • Peripartum • Mental health • Medication • Treatment considerations

KEY POINTS

- Clinicians treating pregnant and postpartum women should be familiar with a range of pharmacologic treatment options, gain comfort with prescribing, and know when to consult a mental health provider.
- Treatment decisions should weigh the risks of medication exposure to fetus or infant with the risks of maternal psychiatric illness on the mother and her family.
- Clinicians should communicate to patients that perinatal depression is a treatable medical condition.

BACKGROUND AND PREVALENCE

Perinatal depression, defined as depressive symptoms occurring either during pregnancy (antenatal depression [AND]) or postpartum (postpartum depression [PPD])[1,2] is exceedingly common and has serious implications when not adequately identified and treated. It has been estimated that between 14% and 23% of women experience AND,[3] and up to 22% of women develop PPD within the first 12 months after delivery.[4] Yet, it has also been estimated that only 30% to 50% of women with AND or PPD are identified in clinical settings, and an even smaller number (14%–16%) receive any treatment for their symptoms.[5]

CONSEQUENCES OF PERINATAL DEPRESSION

Untreated AND has been associated with increased risks for preeclampsia and preterm birth, as well as the development of numerous chronic health complications in

Disclosure Statement: The UNC Department of Psychiatry (S. Meltzer-Brody, M.C. Kimmel) has received research grant support from Sage Therapeutics as a site for their clinical trial of brexanalone. Dr S. Meltzer-Brody has also received research grant support to UNC from Janssen.
Department of Psychiatry, University of North Carolina-Chapel Hill, Campus Box 7160, Chapel Hill, NC 27599-7160, USA
* Corresponding author.
E-mail address: mary_kimmel@med.unc.edu

the mother, including diabetes, hypertension, and cardiovascular disease.[6–8] Furthermore, untreated AND is one of the greatest risk factors for the development of PPD.[3,9,10] Untreated PPD has been associated with unplanned weaning or lactation failure, toxic stress of the newborn, impaired bonding and attachment, and can adversely affect the mental and emotional health of the child through school-age.[11–19] PPD is often a trigger for onset of a chronic major depressive disorder, with almost 1 in 3 women continuing to struggle with depressive symptoms at least 4 years after delivery.[20] Most important, PPD is considered to be the greatest risk factor for maternal suicide and infanticide.[21]

WEIGHING THE RISKS: PSYCHOTROPIC MEDICATION AND PERINATAL DEPRESSION

The American Psychiatric Association and American Congress of Obstetrics and Gynecology both recommend either psychotherapy or antidepressant medication as first-line treatment for mild to moderate perinatal depression.[22] Many women express concern about the effects of medication on the fetus or nursing infant,[23] and prefer psychotherapy as the initial approach to their depressive symptoms.[23,24] Both cognitive–behavioral therapy and interpersonal therapy are efficacious treatments for mild to moderate perinatal depression.[25–27] A recent metaanalysis demonstrated that therapies with an interpersonal component (eg, interpersonal therapy) lead to the greatest reduction in depressive symptoms.[28] Interpersonal therapy is a particularly good fit for addressing perinatal depression given its:

1. Time-limited nature,
2. Goal of positively impacting interpersonal functioning, including the mother–infant relationship and relationship with the husband or partner, and
3. Focus on increasing social support more broadly, which is critically important for maternal well-being.[29]

Psychotherapy during the perinatal period should be delivered individually whenever possible because it leads to greater improvement in depressive symptoms compared with group therapy.[28] Although there have not been any randomized controlled trials (RCTs) of psychotherapy versus pharmacotherapy for perinatal depression, epidemiologic data suggest that, for moderate to severe symptoms, psychotherapy alone may not be sufficient, and augmentation with pharmacotherapy ought to be considered.[30] For those receiving both psychotherapy and pharmacotherapy, a multidisciplinary, integrated care team, including the prescribing physician and therapist, is critical for monitoring symptoms and working collaboratively to address both the psychosocial[31] and biological[32] aspects of perinatal depression.

When considering medication use in pregnancy, the thoughtful weighing of potential risks of untreated depressive symptoms in both the mother and developing baby compared with the risk of medication exposure is needed. No decision is completely risk free and the goal of treatment is minimization of risk with efficacy of treatment. All psychotropic medications cross the placenta and no psychotropic medication is approved by the US Food and Drug Administration (FDA) for use during pregnancy.[33] Given that gold standard RCTs for pregnant women and psychotropic medications are not available, we rely on data from case reports, case control studies, and administrative databases.[30] Potential risks to the fetus that must be considered include teratogenicity and neonatal toxicity and/or withdrawal, as well as long-term effects on development. When medication is required, often the best choice is the drug that previously demonstrated good efficacy for the individual, although this choice must be balanced against the safety of the particular drug during pregnancy. Medication should be titrated to the lowest effective therapeutic dose, with a goal of full symptom remission. As pregnancy progresses, higher doses of psychotropic medication may be required owing to the marked changes in plasma volumes and drug clearance rates during pregnancy. Therefore, collaborative interdisciplinary care among obstetrics, psychiatry, and pediatrics is of utmost importance to ensure the best clinical outcomes.

SELECTIVE SEROTONIN REUPTAKE INHIBITORS, FIRST-LINE PHARMACOLOGIC TREATMENT

Selective serotonin reuptake inhibitors (SSRIs) are usually considered first-line pharmacologic treatment agents for perinatal depression, including both depressive and anxiety symptoms.[34] See **Table 1** for a list of SSRIs and specifics around dosing and unique considerations. SSRIs inhibit the reuptake of serotonin at the synaptic cleft, thereby amplifying serotonin signaling in the brain.[35] Efficacy and tolerability of different SSRIs have been largely similar in clinical trials.[36,37]

Small for Gestational Age, Preterm Delivery, and Spontaneous Abortion

There have been conflicting data about SSRI exposure during pregnancy and the potential risk of small for gestational age, preterm delivery, and spontaneous abortion. These risks have been associated with perinatal depression itself and the risk may lie with the illness rather than exposure.[38–40] Liu and colleagues[41] found that children of women who continued antidepressants were at greater risk of psychiatric disorders than women who discontinued antidepressants during pregnancy. Continuation may be a marker for more severe depression.

Teratogenicity

Most current data looking at exposure to all SSRIs show no consistent information to support specific teratogenic risks.[42]

Persistent Pulmonary Hypertension of the Newborn

Previous studies have reported conflicting data about increased risk of persistent pulmonary hypertension of the newborn (PPHN) with SSRI exposure during pregnancy, leading the FDA to revise their warning in 2011 to state that the risk is inconclusive.[43–45] However, the most up-to-date publication examining a cohort of more than 3 million women, and adjusting for potential confounding variables, concluded a very small increased absolute risk for PPHN with SSRI exposure (adjusted odds ratio of 1.28 for SSRIs vs 1.14 for non-SSRIs).[46]

Neonatal Toxicity and/or Withdrawal

With pregnancy exposure to SSRIs, there has been evidence of increased risk for medication withdrawal or poor neonatal adaptation syndrome (PNAS) at the time of delivery.[47,48] PNAS has been estimated to occur in up to 30% of exposed babies and can manifest as a range of symptoms, including irritability, respiratory distress, hypoglycemia, feeding difficulties, increased or decreased tone, sleep disturbance, and, more rarely, seizures, prolonged QT interval, or cardiac arrhythmias.[47] PNAS can present minutes to hours after birth and typically resolves within 1 to 2 days.[49] If present, PNAS is usually mild and transient, without residual issues. The likelihood of PNAS being more severe and requiring more significant intervention may occur in up to 3% of exposed neonates.[50] Some investigators have hypothesized that PNAS may be related to a neurologic phenomenon, rather than simply toxicity or withdrawal

Table 1
Medications, dosing, and unique considerations

Generic Name	Trade Name	Dosage Range	Unique Considerations/Indications
SSRIs[a]			
Sertraline	Zoloft, Serafem	50–200 mg,[b] increase by 25 mg or 50 mg, for very anxious patients 12.5 mg	Due to half-life small, even negligible amounts transmitted into breast milk.
Fluoxetine	Prozac	20–80 mg, increase by 10 mg or 20 mg	Longer half-life → withdrawal less likely if doses are missed, but also longer to get out of the system if there are adverse effects, likely greater amount in breast milk, thought to be more activating.
Citalopram	Celexa	20–40 mg, increase by 10 mg or 20 mg	FDA Drug Safety Communication that >40 mg could result in a life-threatening heart arrhythmia.
Escitalopram	Lexapro	10–20 mg,[b] increase by 5 mg or 10 mg	
Paroxetine	Paxil, Pexeva, Brisdelle	10–60 mg, increase by 10 mg or 20 mg, CR in 12.5 mg doses	Older data demonstrated potential for a 1.5- to 2.0-fold increase risk in cardiovascular malformations,[141] leading to a 2005 warning.[142] Recent data show no consistent information to support teratogenic risks.[42]
Fluvoxamine	Luvox, Faverin, Fevarin, Floxyfral, Dumyrox	25–150 mg, increase by 25 mg	More often used for treatment of obsessive compulsive disorder.
SNRIs[c]			
Venlafaxine	Effexor, Effexor XR	37.5–375.0 mg, increase by 37.5 mg	Older and most data available.
Duloxetine	Cymbalta, Irenka	20–120 mg, increase by 20 mg, 30 mg	
Milnacipran	Savella	100 mg BID–200 mg, increase by 12.5 mg, 25 mg, 50 mg	No studies currently available on use in pregnancy examining neither teratogenic risks nor available data about long-term developmental outcomes.

Desvenlafaxine	Pristiq, Khedezia	25–400 mg	No studies currently available on use in pregnancy examining neither teratogenic risks nor available data about long-term developmental outcomes. No evidence >50 mg is helpful.
Other antidepressants: Their own unique mechanisms of action			
Buproprion	Wellbutrin SR, Wellbutrin XL, Zyban, Aplenzin, and Forfivo XL	150–450 mg, increase by 150 mg, SR BID dosing	Not to exceed 450 mg owing to an increased risk of seizure, greater concern for seizure in those with a history of seizure or those engaging in purging behaviors. Helpful for smoking cessation[144] and even evidence for lower prematurity risk for smokers.[145] May help ADHD and other addictive disorders, such as overeating.
Mirtazepine	Remeron	15–45 mg, increase by 7.5 mg, 15 mg	Antiemetic effects in addition to antidepressant and anxiolytic effects,[146,147] and helps with sleep and decreased appetite.
Trazodone, nefazodone	Oleptro, Desyrel, Serzone	50–400 mg, ½ tablet (25 mg)–100 mg for sleep	Sleep aid[148] at lower dosages, higher dosages more antidepressant affects. No differences in the rate of major malformations.[93]
Tricyclic TCAs[d]			
Desipramine, nortriptyline	Norpramin, Pamelor, Aventyl	Dose varies for each TCA	Less anticholinergic, so less orthostatic hypotension and constipation, which are common in pregnancy.[149,150]
Amoxapine, imipramine, doxepin, clomipramine, trimipramine, amitriptyline, protriptyline	Asendin, Tofranil, Sinequan, Silenor, Anafranil, Sumontil, Vivactil, Elavil, Vanatrip	Dose varies for each TCA, blood levels are possible to obtain	
MAOIs[e]			
Isocarboxazid, phenelzine, selegiline, tranylcypromine	Marplan, Nardil, Emsam, Parnate	Dose varies for each MAOI	Requires special diet, interacts with some medications to cause life-threatening hypertensive crisis.

(continued on next page)

Table 1
(continued)

Generic Name	Trade Name	Dosage Range	Unique Considerations/Indications
Mood stabilizer and antidepressant			
Lamotrigine	Lamictal	>50 mg, start at 25 mg daily and increase by 25 mg every 2 wk to decrease risk of Stevens-Johnson syndrome	Some evidence to use for augmentation in treatment-resistant depression,[151,152] OCD,[153,154] and, therefore, possibly obsessive compulsive symptoms of perinatal depression,[155] and for mood dysregulation and aggressive behaviors of borderline personality disorder, which is often comorbid with depression.[156]
Atypical antipsychotics (aripiprazole, quetiapine, olanzapine, risperidone, ziprasidone, lurasidone, paliperidone)	Abilify, Seroquel, Zyprexa, Risperdal, Geodon, Latuda, Invega		With augmentation of depression resulted in modest but statistically significant increased likelihood of remission during 12 wk of treatment compared with switching to bupropion monotherapy[157]; small study found less likely to have a postpartum mood episode.[158]
Lithium		Increase by 150 mg, 300 mg; Therapeutic blood level 0.4–0.8 for depression augmentation, 0.8–1.2 for mood stabilization	Helpful for monotherapy and augmentation of unipolar depression,[159,160] and postpartum psychosis in addition to Bipolar Disorder.[161] Increases the likelihood of maintaining mood stability during pregnancy and preventing postpartum relapse[162–164] as does immediately restarting postpartum[162,165]

Abbreviations: ADHD, attention deficit hyperactivity disorder; BID, 2 times per day; CR, controlled release; FDA, US Food and Drug Administration; MAOI, monoamine oxidase inhibitor; OCD, obsessive–compulsive disorder; SNRI, Serotonin norepinephrine reuptake inhibitor; SSRI, selective serotonin reuptake inhibitor; TCA, tricyclic antidepressant; XR, extended release.

[a] All treat depression and anxiety, higher dosages needed for anxiety, Black Box warning for use in children secondary to an increased risk of suicidal thoughts at initiation (still used to treat depression, anxiety, which will decrease risk of suicide), increase dosage for 1 week for menses for premenstrual mood worsening or anxiety.

[b] Some providers may increase to 250 mg or 30 mg.

[c] Treat depression and anxiety, and have also shown to be effective treatments for chronic pain.[143]

[d] First discovered in the 1950s, revolutionized treatment of depression and preceded SSRIs,[88] but are associated with higher mortality rates owing to overdose.[89] Helpful for chronic pain.

[e] Gracious and Wisner[90] indicate a use in patients with atypical depression that have not otherwise responded.

from medication.[51] Importantly, tapering medication to avoid PNAS during the third trimester is not advised, because it has not been shown to improve neonatal health or outcomes, and could place the mother at significant risk of worsened symptoms and decline.[51] Breastfeeding may additionally help to minimize or ease any potential serotonin withdrawal symptoms for the infant in the early postpartum period.[52]

Long-Term Developmental Outcomes

The risk for autism spectrum disorders associated with SSRI exposure during pregnancy is controversial. Maternal depression has been found to be potentially neurotoxic, and is a considerable confounding variable.[53] Some studies have shown potential risk for autism spectrum disorders with SSRI exposure[54–56]; however, when adjusted for confounders, including the risk of maternal depression, statistical significance is usually lost.[57–59] Other developmental outcomes that must be considered with perinatal exposure to psychotropic medications include language, growth, and motor development. Review of available data demonstrates no effects of in utero SSRI exposure on head circumference, weight, or length during the first year of life.[60] Examination of the literature on IQ and behaviors of sibling pairs in mother's with and without SSRI exposure during pregnancy showed that the child's IQ was predicted by maternal IQ. Maternal depression has an impact on problematic behaviors in the children.[53] Last, a longitudinal study of the development in children with in utero SSRI exposure found no differences in mental indices; psychomotor scores were mildly lower during the first year of life, and then normalized thereafter.[61]

SEROTONIN NOREPINEPHRINE REUPTAKE INHIBITORS, IMPORTANT ALTERNATIVES

Serotonin norepinephrine reuptake inhibitors (SNRIs), as detailed in **Table 1**, are important alternatives in the treatment of perinatal depressive and anxiety symptoms especially when nonresponsive to SSRIs or if the patient has previously done well on an SNRI.[62,63] SNRIs have a mixed mechanism of action on both serotonin and norepinephrine and have demonstrated good efficacy for treatment refractory depression[35,64] There are fewer data available for SNRI use during pregnancy than for SSRIs.

There has been 1 study in rats showing potential increased risk for cardiac anomalies with venlafaxine exposure in utero.[65] However, available human data, including an aggregate metaanalysis of multidatabase studies including 2.3 million Nordic births, concluded there was no evidence for venlafaxine-related cardiovascular birth defects.[66] The literature comprises a systematic review from 2016, a separate comprehensive appraisal of 29 available studies in 2015, and a 2001 prospective controlled study of 150 exposures to in utero venlafaxine, all of which failed to find an increased rate of major malformations.[67–69] Although there are fewer data with Duloxetine, available studies to date have not found evidence of an apparent increased risk of congenital malformations.[67,69,70]

Data from the Quebec Pregnancy Cohort between 1998 and 2009 investigating risk between SNRI/SSRI exposure and risk for PPHN did not find a statistically significant association; however, the lack of power for the SNRI arm of the study makes the risk assessment ultimately unclear, because there was a small but significantly increased risk with SSRI exposure during the second half of pregnancy in that study.[71]

There is 1 study examining placental transfer of 2 SSRIs (paroxetine and fluoxetine) and 1 SNRI (venlafaxine), which found no pattern of PNAS association with placental transfer of different antidepressants owing to large interindividual variability for each medication[72] However, as with SSRIs, there is potential increased risk for SNRI toxicity or withdrawal/PNAS. Symptom manifestation and presentation for SNRIs is likely relatively similar.[73] Also, as observed with PNAS management with SSRIs, breastfeeding may help to ease any potential risk for withdrawal symptoms from SNRIs.[73,74]

There are few data available for long-term developmental effects of SNRI exposure in pregnancy. One study examining 62 exposed children ages 3 to 7 years found that IQ was predicted by maternal IQ and not SNRI exposure or duration of SNRI exposure.[53] There is 1 available study looking at desvenlafaxine exposure during pregnancy in Swiss albino mice that found potential risk for increase in anxiety and fearfulness in offspring that could be indicative of possible impact on brain development.[75]

BUPROPION AND MIRTAZAPINE, UNIQUE PROPERTIES

Bupropion inhibits norepinephrine and dopamine reuptake and is the only antidepressant of its kind.[35] The most common side effects are dry mouth, insomnia, and nausea.[76–78] Mirtazapine, a noradrenergic and specific serotonergic antidepressant, has been shown to be comparable with SSRIs in the acute phase treatment of non-pregnancy-related depression.[79,80] See **Table 1** for more on their unique properties and indications.

The literature has been conflicting on risk of bupropion exposure during pregnancy and adverse effects on the fetus. Some studies show no association of first trimester bupropion exposure with congenital or cardiovascular malformations compared with other antidepressants or bupropion exposure outside of the first trimester.[81] Interestingly, the data from this initial report were reanalyzed using more stringent case definitions and concluded that there is a small increased risk, although also acknowledging an inability to account for confounders.[82] Other reports have also shown a positive association between first trimester bupropion use and left outflow tract heart defects, but the magnitude of the observed increased risk was small.[83] More recently, Louik and colleagues[84] in 2014, using data from Slone Epidemiology Center's Case-control Birth Defect Study, concluded that they could not confirm the association with left-sided cardiac defects, but did find an increased risk of ventricular septal defect.

Given this conflicting and relatively small literature, as well as the difficulty accounting for confounders, the risk of bupropion exposure versus nontreatment should be considered carefully, as with any medication in pregnancy. Patients should be counseled that bupropion and its metabolites have been found to cross the placenta,[85] but this should factor be weighed against the risks of depression or smoking for the patient and the baby.

A review of the literature on mirtazapine in pregnancy and lactation included 31 papers with 390 cases of neonates, and concluded that mirtazapine is not associated with increased risk of malformations; however, there was not enough information to make any conclusions on risks of mirtazapine during lactation.[86] Of note, typical exposure through lactation involves even more factors, such as amount in the mother's blood, protein binding and oral bioavailability,[87] which often manifests as reduced transfer to the newborn.

TRICYCLIC ANTIDEPRESSANTS, MONOAMINE OXIDASE INHIBITORS, AND TRAZODONE

Tricyclic antidepressants (TCAs), first discovered in the 1950s, revolutionized the treatment of depression and preceded SSRIs.[88] TCAs are associated with higher mortality rates owing to overdose.[89] Monoamine oxidase inhibitors were also first discovered in the 1950s.[88] There is very little data on monoamine oxidase inhibitors.[90] Trazodone also has limited data. All 3 agents are discussed in **Table 1**. Limb anomalies in earlier studies of TCAs have not been confirmed and neonatal behavioral effects from fetal exposure have not been reported.[91] Monoamine oxidase inhibitors included in a study with other antidepressants did not identify adverse fetal outcomes.[92] A study of 147 women taking nefazadone or trazodone were compared with 2 other groups—women taking other antidepressants or women taking another nonpsychotropic medication thought to be nonteratogenic—and found no differences in the rate of major malformations.[93] Conceivably, the same concerns as for SSRIs may be present, such as for possible increased risk of PPHN.[94] Similar to SSRIs, neonatal symptoms, such as transient withdrawal symptoms, have been reported.[91] TCAs studied in the Quebec Pregnancy Cohort were associated with eye, ear, face, neck, and digestive defects, although the confidence interval for the eye, ear, face, and neck defects was very close to 1.0.[95] Several cohorts of exposed children have been followed with no identified negative neurobehavioral effects of TCAs.[96–98]

AUGMENTATION MEDICATIONS (LITHIUM, ATYPICAL ANTIPSYCHOTICS, AND LAMOTRIGINE)

See **Table 1** for more details about lithium, atypical antipsychotics and lamotrigine used for augmentation. Recent literature has shown that lithium's association with cardiac malformations is smaller than previously thought,[99] and must be weighed against the risks of the illness itself. Although limited, data for lithium and second-generation antipsychotics indicate effects are reassuring with regards to child development.[100] Despite some earlier concerns, subsequent studies have suggested that lamotrigine is not associated with an increased risk of congenital malformations.[101] The long-term safety profile of lamotrigine during pregnancy is promising. In a review that included 8 studies, lamotrigine had no adverse outcomes on infant IQ or neurodevelopment.[102]

NEW DEVELOPMENTS IN DRUG SAFETY LABELING AND MONITORING

This review does not include information on the FDA pregnancy risk categories (A, B, C, D, and X), which began in 1979.[103] This labeling system has been criticized for not adequately reflecting the complexity of decision making about medication use during pregnancy. This system is not conducive to assessing relative risk within categories, has often been viewed as hierarchical rather than descriptive, and does not readily allow for updating based on new findings.[103,104]

In December 2014, the FDA published the Content and Format of Labeling for Human Prescription Drug and Biological Products; Requirements for Pregnancy and Lactation Labeling, also referred to as the "Pregnancy and Lactation Labeling Rule." The rule was implemented on June 30, 2015. It requires medication labels to include a risk summary and clinical considerations, including information relevant for decision making, such as the risk of untreated conditions, complications, and interventions, and data. It prioritizes the inclusion of new information available from drug registries and postmarketing surveillance. Medications approved after 2001 will be required to implement this new labeling by June of 2020, and those approved before 2001, to remove letter ratings by June 30, 2018.[103,105] More information is available at https://www.fda.gov/Drugs/DevelopmentApprovalProcess/DevelopmentResources/Labeling/ucm093307.html.

ESTRADIOL AND PROGESTIN TREATMENTS

Many investigators have hypothesized that alterations in reproductive hormones contribute to PPD because of the temporal association between the precipitous decrease in hormone concentrations that occur with childbirth and the onset of mood symptoms.[106] Reproductive hormones have been shown to play a role in basic emotion processing, arousal, cognition, and motivation, and they regulate each of the biological systems implicated in depression (eg, thyroid, immune, and hypothalamic–pituitary–adrenal axis function and genetic expression).[32] Reproductive hormones also regulate neurotransmitter synthesis, release, and transport, impacting the neural systems implicated in depression.[32] Experimental studies have shown that some women with a history of PPD are differentially sensitive to the effects of changes of estrogen and progesterone on mood.[107] One pilot study of pregnant women with a history of PPD showed that prophylactic administration of oral Premarin, a conjugated estrogen, prevented PPD recurrence in 10 of the 11 women studied.[108] A later double-blind, placebo-controlled trial of 61 women with PPD that began within 3 months after delivery showed that women treated with transdermal estradiol (n = 34) showed a greater decrease in depressive symptoms than those who received placebo (n = 27), although almost one-half of the women in each group were also taking antidepressants.[109] Finally, another study of 23 women with severe PPD, many of whom had not experienced benefit from treatment with either antidepressant medication or psychotherapy, and were found to have low concentrations of serum estradiol, were considered to be in "gonadal failure," and showed symptom remission after 8 weeks of sublingual estrogen treatment.[110] Estradiol may be an effective treatment for PPD; however, a large RCT is needed before recommending hormonal treatment in the postpartum period given the known risks of impaired lactation and venous thromboembolism with oral estrogen preparations. The only large-scale RCT to date was stopped early after finding that treatment with 200 μg transdermal estradiol did not result in significantly increased serum estradiol concentrations.[111] There is even less evidence for progesterone treatment for PPD. One study found norethisterone enanthate, a synthetic progestogen, administered within 48 hours of delivery, was associated with a significantly higher risk of developing PPD.[112] Of note, in a small study of nonpregnant women across the spectrum from anorexia nervosa to normal weight to obese, progesterone levels were not associated with depressive or anxiety symptoms; however, allopregnanolone levels were.[113] Intravenous allopregnanolone therapy is promising and discussed in the Future Directions section.

GENERAL RULES OF THUMB AND TREATMENT ALGORITHM

The rule of thumb for treating perinatal women is that one size does not fit all, and each patient should have an individualized discussion with her provider about the risks of medication weighed against her own risks of not taking medication during pregnancy or lactation. Women who decide they want to come off medications should do so with the supervision of a physician, and ideally preconceptionally. Abrupt medication discontinuation has been associated with high relapse rates. In a prospective sample of 201 euthymic women on stable doses of antidepressants at the time of conception, 68% who discontinued medications during pregnancy experienced relapse of symptoms, and 60% of those who stopped their medication restarted it later in pregnancy.[114] Predictors of relapse included having 4 or more prior depressive episodes and suffering illness for more than 5 years.[114] The most judicious approach is to use the least amount of medication that helps a woman feel better and keeps her well. As noted, it is important to recognize that higher dosages are often required than prepregnancy dosages owing to increased blood volume and increased metabolism during pregnancy. Managing sleep and comorbidities, while providing a multidisciplinary treatment approach, will improve outcomes with medication treatment of perinatal depression.

Breastfeeding is promoted by all major medical groups for the first year of the child's life to improve both maternal and infant health outcomes.[115] Therefore, to minimize stress on the mother, for most medications pumping and dumping (ie, pumping and then throwing out all milk while taking a medication or after taking the medication throwing out the first pump of milk after taking the medication) is not advised[87] However, there may be cases where the risk–benefit ratio supports this practice, such as in the case of a treatment agent that may have high likelihood of passing into breast milk. As noted, the amount of medication exposure in breast milk is thought to be far less than exposure during pregnancy through transplacental passage. Data from the National Institutes of Health have demonstrated that SSRIs are compatible with breastfeeding.[74] It is important to collaborate with the infant's pediatrician when a mother is taking a psychotropic medication during lactation, and to monitor the infant for sedation, proper weight gain, and achievement of developmental milestones. For any medication other than lithium, the literature does not support checking infant blood levels.[116] For questions, an important resource is LACTMED, https://toxnet.nlm.nih.gov/newtoxnet/lactmed.html, a database from the National Institutes of Health, with information on medication patients may have taken during pregnancy.

We have developed a treatment algorithm based on the literature and the clinical experience of our perinatal psychiatry team (**Fig. 1**). For a patient who has not tried medication before, sertraline is a good first choice given it is often well-tolerated, has efficacy for anxiety symptoms along with depressive symptoms, is an older medication with a relatively large evidence base, and has low breast milk concentrations in mother–infant dyad studies.[116] In general, medications that are less lipophilic, with shorter half-lives, are less likely to cross the placenta or cross into breast milk. However, if a patient is doing well with, or has done well with, another type of antidepressant, then it is better to continue with that medication, especially if other medications have not been effective for the patient. Alternatively, if a patient is not responding to a medication, it is important to consider other complicating factors and rethink the diagnosis. For STAR*D participants with major depression (general outpatients including men and women ages 18–75), severity, poor treatment adherence, and poor physical health increased the risk of depression failing to, or taking a longer time to remit. Social factors such as unemployment was also associated with nonremission.[117] Clinicians must also carefully screen for history of mania or hypomania to rule out bipolar spectrum illness, as a different treatment algorithm should then be applied, and antidepressants could significantly worsen symptoms if used alone.[2,35,118,119] Those presenting with first episodes of depression in the postpartum period are more likely to develop bipolar affective disorder and psychotic symptoms.[120] In addition, those with bipolar disorders I or II are associated with PPD rates as high as 50%.[121] The psychosis specifier of major depressive disorder is found more often in women who are postpartum than in those with depressive episodes during pregnancy, as well as nonpregnant women.[122,123] Psychotic symptoms can sometimes be hard to gather, so spending some time talking with patients and with their family and supports will help to identify those symptoms. If there is a question of psychosis, emergency referral to perinatal psychiatry is important.

FUTURE DIRECTIONS FOR PHARMACOLOGIC TREATMENT OF PERINATAL DEPRESSION

There is new evidence that the neurosteroid, allopregnanolone, a major metabolite of progesterone, may potentially contribute to the etiology and treatment of PPD.[32,124] Allopregnolone is a positive allosteric modulator of synaptic and extrasynaptic GABA-A receptors[125,126] and animal models have demonstrated that it has significant

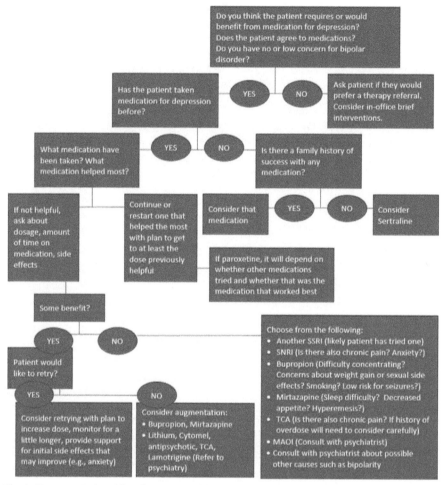

Fig. 1. Treatment algorithm for perinatal depression. MAOI, monoamine oxidase inhibitor; SSRI, selective serotonin reuptake inhibitor; TCA, tricyclic antidepressant.

effects on anxiety and depression.[32] Allopregnanolone concentrations rapidly decrease after childbirth, after reaching peak physiologic levels in the third trimester of pregnancy.[32,124] It is hypothesized that the failure of GABA-A receptors to adapt to the rapid fluctuations at childbirth may be a trigger for PPD.[127–130] This line of inquiry is being explored by the development of brexanolone, a proprietary formulation of allopregnanolone as a treatment for PPD. A positive small open-label trial,[131] and more recently, a positive phase II RCT of brexanolone showed rapid and clinically meaningful reductions in depressive symptoms as compared with placebo.[132] Sage Therapeutics (Cambridge, MA) announced in November 2017 that they obtained statistically significant mean reduction depressive symptoms with brexanolone compared with placebo at 60 hours, and was durable over 30 days in 2 placebo-controlled multicenter phase III trials.[133]

Another possible novel area of intervention may be the microbiota–gut–brain axis. Preliminary findings from an RCT testing the use of a probiotics in pregnancy warrant further study with regard to depressive and anxiety symptoms.[134,135] Although there is no evidence as of yet to support the use of probiotic pills, the gut microbiota may be an important mediator of antidepressant effects given that certain microbes are involved in tryptophan and serotonin metabolism, and in drug metabolism.[136,137] Additional microbiome research may allow for better understanding of how medications are metabolized and best used during the perinatal period.

There is great need for innovative models regarding delivery of care to perinatal women. The literature demonstrates that only a small percentage of perinatal women are adequately screened and treated for perinatal depression[5,138] owing to multiple barriers.[139] Integrated care models that embed mental health providers in obstetric settings and specialized perinatal psychiatry inpatient units may further ensure patients better access and care.[140]

SUMMARY

Perinatal depression is a treatable medical condition. There are many evidence-based treatments, but novel treatment paradigms are also needed to target the underlying pathogenesis of perinatal depression and to increase the efficacy of treatment. Treatment can have important reductions in suffering for women and their families.

REFERENCES

1. World Health Organisation. ICD-10 classifications of mental and behavioural disorder: clinical descriptions and diagnostic guidelines. 1992.
2. American Psychiatric Association. Diagnostic and statistical manual of mental disorders. 5th edition. Arlington (VA): American Psychiatric Publishing; 2013.
3. Gaynes B, Gavin N, Meltzer-Brody S. Perinatal depression: prevalence, screening accuracy and screening outcomes. Evid Rep Technol Assess 2005; 119:1–8.
4. Elisei S, Lucarini E, Murgia N, et al. Perinatal depression: a study of prevalence and of risk and protective factors. Psychiatr Danub 2013;25:S258–62.
5. Cox EQ, Sowa NA, Meltzer-Brody SE, et al. The perinatal depression treatment cascade: baby steps toward improving outcomes. J Clin Psychiatry 2016;77(9): 1189–200.
6. Grigoriadis S, VonderPorten EH, Mamisashvili L, et al. The impact of maternal depression during pregnancy on perinatal outcomes: a systematic review and meta-analysis. J Clin Psychiatry 2013;74(4):321–41.
7. Herring SJ, Rich-Edwards JW, Oken E, et al. Association of postpartum depression with weight retention 1 year after childbirth. Obesity 2008;16:1296–301.
8. Qiu C, Williams MA, Calderon-Margalit R, et al. Preeclampsia risk in relation to maternal mood and anxiety disorders diagnosed before or during early pregnancy. Am J Hypertens 2009;22:397–402.
9. Meltzer-Brody S, Bledsoe-Mansori SE, Johnson N, et al. A prospective study of perinatal depression and trauma history in pregnant minority adolescents. Am J Obstet Gynecol 2013;208(211):e1–7.
10. Milgrom J, Gemmill AW, Bilszta JL, et al. Antenatal risk factors for postnatal depression: a large prospective study. J Affect Disord 2008;108:147–57.
11. Garner AS, Shonkoff JP, Committee on Psychosocial Aspects of Child and Family Health, Committee on Early Childhood, Adoption, and Dependent Care, Section on Developmental and Behavioral Pediatrics. Early childhood adversity, toxic stress, and the role of the pediatrician: translating developmental science into lifelong health. Pediatrics 2012;129(1):e224–31.

12. Earls MF, T.C.o.P.A.o.C.a.F. Health. Clinical report – Incorporating recognition and management of perinatal and postpartum depression into pediatric practice American Academy of Pediatrics, 2010.

13. Shonkoff JP, Garner AS, Committee on Psychosocial Aspects of Child and Family Health, Committee on Early Childhood, Adoption, and Dependent Care, Section on Developmental and Behavioral Pediatrics. The lifelong effects of early childhood adversity and toxic stress. Pediatrics 2012;129(1):e232–46.

14. National Scientific Council on the Developing Child, Center on the Developing Child at Harvard University. Excessive stress disrupts the architecture of the developing brain: paper #3. Cambridge (MA): National Scientific Council on the Developing Child, Center on the Developing Child at Harvard University; 2005.

15. National Scientific Council on the Developing Child. Early Experiences Can Alter Gene Expression and Affect Long-Term Development: Working Paper #10 2010. Available at: http://www.developingchild.net.

16. Dawson G, Ashman S. On the origins of a vulnerability to depression: the influence of the early social environment on the development of psychobiological systems related to risk for affective disorder. In: Nelson C, editor. The effects of adversity on neurobehavioral development: Minnesota symposium on child psychology. Mahwah (NJ): Lawrence Erlbaum & Assoc; 2000. p. 245–80.

17. Ashman S, Dawson G, Panagiotides H, et al. Stress hormone levels of children of depressed mothers. Dev Psychopathol 2002;14(2):333–49.

18. Essex MJ, Klein MH, Cho E, et al. Maternal stress beginning in infancy may sensitize children to later stress exposure: effects on cortisol and behavior. Biol Psychiatry 2002;52(8):776–84.

19. Dennis C, McQueen K. The relationship between infant-feeding outcomes and postpartum depression: a qualitative systematic review. Pediatrics 2009; 123(4):736–51.

20. Woolhouse H, Gartland D, Mensah F, et al. Maternal depression from early pregnancy to 4 years postpartum in a prospective pregnancy cohort study: implications for primary health care. BJOG 2014. https://doi.org/10.1111/1471-0528. 12837.

21. Lindahl V, Pearson J, Colpe L. Prevalence of suicidality during pregnancy and postpartum. Arch Womens Ment Health 2005;8(2):77–87.

22. Yonkers KA, Wisner KL, Stewart DE, et al. The management of depression during pregnancy: a report from the American Psychiatric Association and the American College of Obstetricians and Gynecologists. Gen Hosp Psychiatry 2009;31:403–13.

23. Battle CL, Salisbury AL, Schofield CA, et al. Perinatal antidepressant use: understanding women's preferences and concerns. J Psychiatr Pract 2013;19(6): 443–53.

24. Goodman JH. Women's attitudes, preferences, and perceived barriers to treatment for perinatal depression. Birth 2009;36(1):60–9.

25. Claridge AM. Efficacy of systematically oriented psychotherapies in the treatment of perinatal depression: a meta analysis. Arch Womens Ment Health 2014;17:3–15.

26. Grote NK, Swartz HA, Geibel SL, et al. A randomized controlled trial of culturally relevant, brief interpersonal psychotherapy for perinatal depression. Psychiatr Serv 2009;60(3):313–21.

27. Spinelli MG, Endicott J, Leon AC, et al. A controlled clinical treatment trial of interpersonal psychotherapy for depressed pregnant women at 3 New York City sites. J Clin Psychiatry 2013;74(4):393–9.

28. Sockol LE, Epperson CN, Barber JP. A meta-analysis of treatments for perinatal depression. Clin Psychol Rev 2011;31(5):839–49.

29. O'Hara MW, McCabe JE. Postpartum depression: current status and future directions. Annu Rev Clin Psychol 2013;9:379–407.

30. Wisner KL, Zarin DA, Holmboe ES, et al. Risk-benefit decision making for treatment of depression during pregnancy. Am J Psychiatry 2000;157(12):1933–40.

31. O'Hara M, Swain AW. Rates and risk of postpartum depression-a meta-analysis. Int Rev Psychiatry 1996;8(1):37–54.

32. Schiller CE, Meltzer-Brody S, Rubinow DR. The role of reproductive hormones in postpartum depression. CNS Spectr 2015;20(1):48–59.

33. FDA, Medication Guides, 2017, U.S. Department of Health and Human Services.

34. Weisskopf E, Fischer CJ, Bickle Graz M, et al. Risk-benefit balance assessment of SSRI antidepressant use during pregnancy and lactation based on best available evidence. Expert Opin Drug Saf 2015;14(3):413–27.

35. Mann J. The medical management of depression. N Engl J Med 2005;353(17): 1819–34.

36. Kroenke K, West SL, Swindle R. Similar effectiveness of paroxetine, fluoxetine, and sertraline in primary care: a randomized trial. JAMA 2001;286:2947–55.

37. Stahl S. Placebo-controlled comparison of the selective serotonin reuptake inhibitors citalopram and sertraline. Biol Psychiatry 2000;48:894–901.

38. Huybrechts KF, Sanghani RS, Avorn J, et al. Preterm birth and antidepressant medication use during pregnancy: a systematic review and meta-analysis. PLoS One 2014;9(3):e92778.

39. Andersen JT, Andersen NL, Horwitz H, et al. Exposure to selective serotonin reuptake inhibitors in early pregnancy and the risk of miscarriage. Obstet Gynecol 2014;124(4):655–61.

40. Sujan AC, Rickert ME, Oberg AS, et al. Associations of maternal antidepressant use during the first trimester of pregnancy with preterm birth, small for gestational age, autism spectrum disorder, and attention-deficit/hyperactivity disorder in offspring. JAMA 2017;317(15):1553–62.

41. Liu X, Agerbo E, Ingstrup KG, et al. Antidepressant use during pregnancy and psychiatric disorders in offspring: Danish nationwide register based cohort study. BMJ 2017;358:j3668.

42. Huybrechts KF, Palmsten K, Avorn J, et al. Antidepressant use in pregnancy and the risk of cardiac defects. N Engl J Med 2014;370(25):2397–407.

43. Chambers CD, Hernandez-Diaz S, Van Marter LJ, et al. Selective serotonin-reuptake inhibitors and risk of persistent pulmonary hypertension of the newborn. N Engl J Med 2006;354(6):579–87.

44. Wilson KL, Zelig CM, Harvey JP, et al. Persistent pulmonary hypertension of the newborn is associated with mode of delivery and not with maternal use of selective serotonin reuptake inhibitors. Am J Perinatol 2011;28(1):19–24.

45. US Food and Drug Administration (FDA). FDA Drug Safety Communication: Selective serotonin reuptake inhibitor (SSRI) antidepressant use during pregnancy and reports of a rare heart and lung condition in newborn babies. 2011. Available at: https://http://www.fda.gov/Drugs/DrugSafety/ucm283375.htm. Accessed October 20, 2017.

46. Huybrechts KF, Bateman BT, Palmsten K, et al. Antidepressant use in late pregnancy and risk of persistent pulmonary hypertension of the newborn. JAMA 2015;313(21):2142–51.

47. Levinson-Castiel R, Merlob P, Linder N, et al. Neonatal abstinence syndrome after in utero exposure to selective serotonin reuptake inhibitors in term infants. Arch Pediatr Adolesc Med 2006;160(2):173–6.

48. Oberlander TF, Misri S, Fitzgerald CE, et al. Pharmacologic factors associated with transient neonatal symptoms following prenatal psychotropic medication exposure. J Clin Psychiatry 2004;65(2):230–7.

49. Moses-Kolko EL, Bogen D, Perel J, et al. Neonatal signs after late in utero exposure to serotonin reuptake inhibitors: literature review and implications for clinical applications. JAMA 2005;293(19):2372–83.

50. Forsberg L, Navér L, Gustafsson LL, et al. Neonatal adaptation in infants prenatally exposed to antidepressants- clinical monitoring using neonatal abstinence score. PLoS One 2014;9(11):e111327.

51. Warburton W, Hertzman C, Oberlander TF. A register study of the impact of stopping third trimester selective serotonin reuptake inhibitor exposure on neonatal health. Acta Psychiatr Scand 2010;121(6):471–9.

52. Kieviet N, Dolman KM, Honig A. The use of psychotropic medication during pregnancy: how about the newborn? Neuropsychiatr Dis Treat 2013;9:1257–66.

53. Nulman I, Koren G, Rovet J, et al. Neurodevelopment of children prenatally exposed to selective reuptake inhibitor antidepressants: Toronto sibling study. J Clin Psychiatry 2015;76(7):e842–7.

54. Croen LA, Grether JK, Yoshida CK, et al. Antidepressant use during pregnancy and childhood autism spectrum disorders. Arch Gen Psychiatry 2011;68(11): 1104–12.

55. Rai D, Lee BK, Dalman C, et al. Parental depression, maternal antidepressant use during pregnancy, and the risk of autism spectrum disorders: population based case-control study. BMJ 2013;346:f2059.

56. Boukhris T, Sheehy O, Mottron L, et al. Antidepressant use during pregnancy and the risk of autism spectrum disorder in children. JAMA Pediatr 2016; 170(2):117–24.

57. Andrade C. Antidepressant exposure during pregnancy and risk of autism in the offspring, 1: meta-review of meta-analyses. J Clin Psychiatry 2017;78(8): e1047–51.

58. Castro VM, Kong SW, Clements CC, et al. Absence of evidence for increase in risk for autism or attention-deficit hyperactivity disorder following antidepressant exposure during pregnancy: a replication study. Transl Psychiatry 2016;6:e708.

59. Oberlander TF, Gingrich JA, Ansorge MS. Sustained neurobehavioral effects of exposure to SSRI antidepressants during development: molecular to clinical evidence. Clin Pharmacol Ther 2009;86(6):672–7.

60. Wisner KL, Bogen DL, Sit D, et al. Does fetal exposure to SSRIs or maternal depression impact infant growth? Am J Psychiatry 2013;170(5):485–93.

61. Santucci AK, Singer LT, Wisniewski SR, et al. Impact of prenatal exposure to serotonin reuptake inhibitors or maternal major depressive disorder on infant developmental outcomes. J Clin Psychiatry 2014;75(10):1088–95.

62. Rush A, Fava M, Wisniewski SR, et al. Sequenced treatment alternatives to relieve depression (STAR*D): rationale and design. Control Clin Trials 2004; 25(1):119–42.

63. Gaynes BN, Warden D, Trivedi MH, et al. What did STAR*D teach us? Results from a large-scale, practical, clinical trial for patients with depression. Psychiatr Serv 2009;60(11):1439–45.
64. Lambert O, Bourin M. SNRIs: mechanism of action and clinical features. Expert Rev Neurother 2002;2(6):849–58.
65. Laurent L, Huang C, Ernest SR, et al. In utero exposure to venlafaxine, a serotonin-norepinephrine reuptake inhibitor, increases cardiac anomalies and alters placental and heart serotonin signaling in the rat. Birth Defects Res A Clin Mol Teratol 2016;106(12):1044–55.
66. Selmer R, Haglund B, Furu K, et al. Individual-based versus aggregate meta-analysis in multi-database studies of pregnancy outcomes: the Nordic example of selective serotonin reuptake inhibitors and venlafaxine in pregnancy. Pharmacoepidemiol Drug Saf 2016;25(10):1160–9.
67. Bellantuono C, Vargas M, Mandarelli G, et al. The safety of serotonin-noradrenaline reuptake inhibitors (SNRIs) in pregnancy and breastfeeding: a comprehensive review. Hum Psychopharmacol 2015;30(3):143–51.
68. Einarson A, Fatoye B, Sarkar M, et al. Pregnancy outcome following gestational exposure to venlafaxine: a multicenter prospective controlled study. Am J Psychiatry 2001;158(10):1728–30.
69. Lassen D, Ennis ZN, Damkier P. First-trimester pregnancy exposure to venlafaxine or duloxetine and risk of major congenital malformations: a systematic review. Basic Clin Pharmacol Toxicol 2016;118(1):32–6.
70. Einarson A, Smart K, Vial T, et al. Rates of major malformations in infants following exposure to duloxetine during pregnancy: a preliminary report. J Clin Psychiatry 2012;73(11):1471.
71. Berard A, Sheehy O, Zhao JP, et al. SSRI and SNRI use during pregnancy and the risk of persistent pulmonary hypertension of the newborn. Br J Clin Pharmacol 2017;83(5):1126–33.
72. Ewing G, Tatarchuk Y, Appleby D, et al. Placental transfer of antidepressant medications: implications for postnatal adaptation syndrome. Clin Pharmacokinet 2015;54(4):359–70.
73. Holland J, Brown R. Neonatal venlafaxine discontinuation syndrome: a mini-review. Eur J Paediatr Neurol 2017;21(2):264–8.
74. National Institutes of Health. TOXNET Toxicology Data Network. Available at: https://toxnet.nlm.nih.gov. Accessed October 20, 2017.
75. Kumari A, Singh M, Trigunayat A, et al. Prenatal desvenlafaxine induced behavioral alterations in Swiss albino mice. Ann Neurosci 2014;21(1):19–21.
76. Anthenelli RM, Benowitz NL, West R, et al. Neuropsychiatric safety and efficacy of varenicline, bupropion, and nicotine patch in smokers with and without psychiatric disorders (EAGLES): a double-blind, randomised, placebo-controlled clinical trial. Lancet 2016;387(10037):2507–20.
77. Hughes JR, Stead LF, Hartmann-Boyce J, et al. Antidepressants for smoking cessation. Cochrane Database Syst Rev 2014;(1):CD000031.
78. Baraona LK, Lovelace D, Daniels JL, et al. Tobacco harms, nicotine pharmacology, and pharmacologic tobacco cessation interventions for women. J Midwifery Womens Health 2017;62(3):253–69.
79. Anttila SA, Leinonen EV. A review of the pharmacological and clinical profile of mirtazapine. CNS Drug Rev 2001;7(3):249–64.
80. Watanabe N, Omori IM, Nakagawa A, et al. Mirtazapine versus other antidepressive agents for depression. Cochrane Database Syst Rev 2011;(12):CD006528.

81. Cole JA, Modell JG, Haight BR, et al. Bupropion in pregnancy and the prevalence of congenital malformations. Pharmacoepidemiol Drug Saf 2007;16(5): 474–84.

82. Thyagarajan V, Robin Clifford C, Wurst KE, et al. Bupropion therapy in pregnancy and the occurrence of cardiovascular malformations in infants. Pharmacoepidemiol Drug Saf 2012;21(11):1240–2.

83. Alwan S, Reefhuis J, Botto LD, et al. Maternal use of bupropion and risk for congenital heart defects. Am J Obstet Gynecol 2010;203(1):52.e1-6.

84. Louik C, Kerr S, Mitchell AA. First-trimester exposure to bupropion and risk of cardiac malformations. Pharmacoepidemiol Drug Saf 2014;23(10):1066–75.

85. Fokina VM, West H, Oncken C, et al. Bupropion therapy during pregnancy: the drug and its major metabolites in umbilical cord plasma and amniotic fluid. Am J Obstet Gynecol 2016;215(4):497.e1-7.

86. Smit M, Dolman KM, Honig A. Mirtazapine in pregnancy and lactation - A systematic review. Eur Neuropsychopharmacol 2016;26(1):126–35.

87. Burkey BW, Holmes AP. Evaluating medication use in pregnancy and lactation: what every pharmacist should know. J Pediatr Pharmacol Ther 2013;18(3): 247–58.

88. Lopez-Munoz F, Alamo C. Monoaminergic neurotransmission: the history of the discovery of antidepressants from 1950s until today. Curr Pharm Des 2009; 15(14):1563–86.

89. Carvalho AF, Sharma MS, Brunoni AR, et al. The safety, tolerability and risks associated with the use of newer generation antidepressant drugs: a critical review of the literature. Psychother Psychosom 2016;85(5):270–88.

90. Gracious BL, Wisner KL. Phenelzine use throughout pregnancy and the puerperium: case report, review of the literature, and management recommendations. Depress Anxiety 1997;6(3):124–8.

91. ACOG Committee on Practice Bulletins–Obstetrics. ACOG Practice Bulletin: clinical management guidelines for obstetrician-gynecologists number 92, April 2008 (replaces practice bulletin number 87, November 2007). Use of psychiatric medications during pregnancy and lactation. Obstet Gynecol 2008;111(4): 1001–20.

92. Ramos E, St-André M, Rey E, et al. Duration of antidepressant use during pregnancy and risk of major congenital malformations. Br J Psychiatry 2008;192(5): 344–50.

93. Einarson A, Bonari L, Voyer-Lavigne S, et al. A multicentre prospective controlled study to determine the safety of trazodone and nefazodone use during pregnancy. Can J Psychiatry 2003;48(2):106–10.

94. Ram D, Gandotra S. Antidepressants, anxiolytics, and hypnotics in pregnancy and lactation. Indian J Psychiatry 2015;57(Suppl 2):S354–71.

95. Berard A, Zhao JP, Sheehy O. Antidepressant use during pregnancy and the risk of major congenital malformations in a cohort of depressed pregnant women: an updated analysis of the Quebec Pregnancy Cohort. BMJ Open 2017;7(1):e013372.

96. Nulman I, Rovet J, Stewart DE, et al. Neurodevelopment of children exposed in utero to antidepressant drugs. N Engl J Med 1997;336(4):258–62.

97. Nulman I, Rovet J, Stewart DE, et al. Child development following exposure to tricyclic antidepressants or fluoxetine throughout fetal life: a prospective, controlled study. Am J Psychiatry 2002;159(11):1889–95.

98. Simon GE, Cunningham ML, Davis RL. Outcomes of prenatal antidepressant exposure. Am J Psychiatry 2002;159(12):2055–61.

99. Patorno E, Huybrechts KF, Bateman BT, et al. Lithium use in pregnancy and the risk of cardiac malformations. N Engl J Med 2017;376(23):2245–54.

100. Haskey C, Galbally M. Mood stabilizers in pregnancy and child developmental outcomes: a systematic review. Aust N Z J Psychiatry 2017;51(11):1087–97.

101. Bromley RL, Weston J, Marson AG. Maternal use of antiepileptic agents during pregnancy and major congenital malformations in children. JAMA 2017;318(17):1700–1.

102. Ornoy A, Weinstein-Fudim L, Ergaz Z. Antidepressants, antipsychotics, and mood stabilizers in pregnancy: what do we know and how should we treat pregnant women with depression. Birth Defects Res 2017;109(12):933–56.

103. Ramoz LL, Patel-Shori NM. Recent changes in pregnancy and lactation labeling: retirement of risk categories. Pharmacotherapy 2014;34(4):389–95.

104. Dinatale M, Sahin L, Johnson T, et al. Medication use during pregnancy and lactation: introducing the pregnancy and lactation labeling rule. Pediatr Allergy Immunol Pulmonol 2017;30(2):132–4.

105. Whyte J. FDA implements new labeling for medications used during pregnancy and lactation. Am Fam Physician 2016;94(1):12–5.

106. O'Hara MW, Schlechte JA, Lewis DA, et al. Controlled prospective study of postpartum mood disorders: psychological, environmental, and hormonal variables. J Abnorm Psychol 1991;100(1):63–73.

107. Bloch M, Schmidt PJ, Danaceau M, et al. Effects of gonadal steroids in women with a history of postpartum depression. Am J Psychiatry 2000;157(6):924–30.

108. Sichel DA, Cohen LS, Robertson LM, et al. Prophylactic estrogen in recurrent postpartum affective disorder. Biol Psychiatry 1995;38(12):814–8.

109. Gregoire AJ, Kumar R, Everitt B, et al. Transdermal oestrogen for treatment of severe postnatal depression. Lancet 1996;347(9006):930–3.

110. Ahokas A, Kaukoranta J, Wahlbeck K, et al. Estrogen deficiency in severe postpartum depression: successful treatment with sublingual physiologic 17beta-estradiol: a preliminary study. J Clin Psychiatry 2001;62(5):332–6.

111. Wisner KL, Sit DK, Moses-Kolko EL, et al. Transdermal estradiol treatment for postpartum depression: a pilot, randomized trial. J Clin Psychopharmacol 2015;35(4):389–95.

112. Lawrie TA, Hofmeyr GJ, De Jager M, et al. A double-blind randomised placebo controlled trial of postnatal norethisterone enanthate: the effect on postnatal depression and serum hormones. Br J Obstet Gynaecol 1998;105(10):1082–90.

113. Dichtel LE, Lawson EA, Schorr M, et al. Neuroactive steroids and affective symptoms in women across the weight spectrum. Neuropsychopharmacology 2018;43(6):1436–44.

114. Cohen LS, Altshuler LL, Harlow BL, et al. Relapse of major depression during pregnancy in women who maintain or discontinue antidepressant treatment. JAMA 2006;295(5):499–508.

115. Section on Breastfeeding. Breastfeeding and the use of human milk. Pediatrics 2012;129(3):e827–41.

116. Pinheiro E, Bogen DL, Hoxha D, et al. Sertraline and breastfeeding: review and meta-analysis. Arch Womens Ment Health 2015;18(2):139–46.

117. Mojtabai R. Nonremission and time to remission among remitters in major depressive disorder: revisiting STAR*D. Depress Anxiety 2017;34(12):1123–33.

118. First MB, Spitzer RL, Gibbon M, et al. Structured clinical interview for DSM-IV-TR axis I disorders, research version, non-patient edition (SCID-I/NP). New York: N.Y.S.P.I. Biometrics Research; 2002.

119. Patel R, Reiss P, Shetty H, et al. Do antidepressants increase the risk of mania and bipolar disorder in people with depression? A retrospective electronic case register cohort study. BMJ 2015;5(12):e008341.

120. Azorin JM, Angst J, Gamma A, et al. Identifying features of bipolarity in patients with first-episode postpartum depression: findings from the international BRIDGE study. J Affect Disord 2012;136(3):710–5.

121. Mandelli L, Souery D, Bartova L, et al. Bipolar II disorder as a risk factor for postpartum depression. J Affect Disord 2016;204:54–8.

122. Altemus M, Neeb CC, Davis A, et al. Phenotypic differences between pregnancy-onset and postpartum-onset major depressive disorder. J Clin Psychiatry 2012;73(12):e1485–91.

123. Dean C, Kendell RE. The symptomatology of puerperal illnesses. Br J Psychiatry 1981;139:128–33.

124. Epperson CN, Gueorguieva R, Czarkowski KA, et al. Preliminary evidence of reduced occipital GABA concentrations in puerperal women: a 1H-MRS study. Psychopharmacology (Berl) 2006;186(3):425–33.

125. Paul SM, Purdy RH. Neuroactive steroids. FASEB J 1992;6(6):2311–22.

126. Majewska MD, Harrison NL, Schwartz RD, et al. Steroid hormone metabolites are barbiturate-like modulators of the GABA receptor. Science 1986;232(4753):1004–7.

127. Deligiannidis KM, Kroll-Desrosiers AR, Mo S, et al. Peripartum neuroactive steroid and γ-aminobutyric acid profiles in women at-risk for postpartum depression. Psychoneuroendocrinology 2016;70:98–107.

128. Nappi RE, Petraglia F, Luisi S, et al. Serum allopregnanolone in women with postpartum "blues". Obstet Gynecol 2001;97(1):77–80.

129. Luisi S, Petraglia F, Benedetto C, et al. Serum allopregnanolone levels in pregnant women: changes during pregnancy, at delivery, and in hypertensive patients. J Clin Endocrinol Metab 2000;85(7):2429–33.

130. Maguire J, Mody I. GABA(A)R plasticity during pregnancy: relevance to postpartum depression. Neuron 2008;59(2):207–13.

131. Kanes SJ, Colquhoun H, Doherty J, et al. Open-label, proof-of-concept study of brexanolone in the treatment of severe postpartum depression. Hum Psychopharmacol 2017;32(2):e2576, 1–6.

132. Kanes S, Colquhoun H, Gunduz-Bruce H, et al. Brexanolone (SAGE-547 injection) in post-partum depression: a randomised controlled trial. Lancet 2017;390(10093):480–9.

133. Sage therapeutics announces brexanolone achieves primary endpoints in both phase 3 clinical trials in postpartum depression. 2017. Available at: http://investor.sagerx.com/news-releases/news-release-details/sage-therapeutics-announces-brexanolone-achieves-primary. Accessed October 20, 2017.

134. Barthow C, Wickens K, Stanley T, et al. The Probiotics in Pregnancy Study (PiP Study): rationale and design of a double-blind randomised controlled trial to improve maternal health during pregnancy and prevent infant eczema and allergy. BMC Pregnancy Childbirth 2016;16(1):133.

135. Slykerman RF, Hood F, Wickens K, et al. Effect of lactobacillus rhamnosus HN001 in pregnancy on postpartum symptoms of depression and anxiety: a randomised double-blind placebo-controlled trial. EBioMedicine 2017;24:159–65.

136. O'Mahony SM, Clarke G, Borre YE, et al. Serotonin, tryptophan metabolism and the brain-gut-microbiome axis. Behav Brain Res 2015;277:32–48.

137. Gimenez-Bastida JA, Martinez Carreras L, Moya-Pérez A, et al. Pharmacological efficacy/toxicity of drugs: a comprehensive update about the dynamic interplay of microbes. J Pharm Sci 2018;107(3):778–84.

138. Fonseca A, Gorayeb R, Canavarro MC. Womens help-seeking behaviours for depressive symptoms during the perinatal period: socio-demographic and clinical correlates and perceived barriers to seeking professional help. Midwifery 2015;31(12):1177–85.

139. Bayrampour H, McNeil DA, Benzies K, et al. A qualitative inquiry on pregnant women's preferences for mental health screening. BMC Pregnancy Childbirth 2017;17(1):339.

140. Cox EQ, Raines C, Kimmel M, et al. Comprehensive integrated care model to improve maternal mental health. J Obstet Gynecol Neonatal Nurs 2017;46(6): 923–30.

141. GlaxoSmithKline. New safety information regarding paroxetine: findings suggest increased risk over other antidepressants, of congenital malformations, following first trimester exposure to paroxetine. Mississauga (Canada): GlaxoSmithKline; 2005.

142. Laughren T. Approval package for: application number NDA 20-031/S052. FDA; 2006.

143. Rowbotham MC, Goli V, Kunz NR, et al. Venlafaxine extended release in the treatment of painful diabetic neuropathy: a double-blind, placebo-controlled study. Pain 2004;110:697–706.

144. Nanovskaya TN, Oncken C, Fokina VM, et al. Bupropion sustained release for pregnant smokers: a randomized, placebo-controlled trial. Am J Obstet Gynecol 2017;216(4):420.e1–9.

145. Berard A, Zhao JP, O Sheehy. Success of smoking cessation interventions during pregnancy. Am J Obstet Gynecol 2016;215(5):611.e1-8.

146. Abramowitz A, Miller ES, Wisner KL. Treatment options for hyperemesis gravidarum. Arch Womens Ment Health 2017;20(3):363–72.

147. Omay O, Einarson A. Is mirtazapine an effective treatment for nausea and vomiting of pregnancy? A case series. J Clin Psychopharmacol 2017;37(2):260–1.

148. Khazaie H, Ghadami MR, Knight DC, et al. Insomnia treatment in the third trimester of pregnancy reduces postpartum depression symptoms: a randomized clinical trial. Psychiatry Res 2013;210(3):901–5.

149. Wichman CL, Stern TA. Diagnosing and treating depression during pregnancy. Prim Care Companion CNS Disord 2015;17(2):1–11.

150. Nonacs R, Cohen LS. Assessment and treatment of depression during pregnancy: an update. Psychiatr Clin North Am 2003;26(3):547–62.

151. Rihmer Z, Gonda X, Rihmer A, et al. Antidepressant-resistant depression and the bipolar spectrum – diagnostic and therapeutic considerations. Psychiatr Hung 2016;31(2):157–68 [in Hungarian].

152. Barbee JG, Thompson TR, Jamhour NJ, et al. A double-blind placebo-controlled trial of lamotrigine as an antidepressant augmentation agent in treatment-refractory unipolar depression. J Clin Psychiatry 2011;72(10): 1405–12.

153. Bruno A, Micò U, Pandolfo G, et al. Lamotrigine augmentation of serotonin reuptake inhibitors in treatment-resistant obsessive-compulsive disorder: a double-blind, placebo-controlled study. J Psychopharmacol 2012;26(11):1456–62.

154. Khalkhali M, Aram S, Zarrabi H, et al. Lamotrigine augmentation versus placebo in serotonin reuptake inhibitors-resistant obsessive-compulsive disorder: a randomized controlled trial. Iran J Psychiatry 2016;11(2):104–14.

155. O'Hara MW, Wisner KL. Perinatal mental illness: definition, description and aetiology. Best Pract Res Clin Obstet Gynaecol 2014;28(1):3–12.

156. Naguy A, Al-Enezi N. Lamotrigine uses in psychiatric practice-beyond bipolar prophylaxis a hope or hype? Am J Ther 2017. [Epub ahead of print].

157. Mohamed S, Johnson GR, Chen P, et al. Effect of antidepressant switching vs augmentation on remission among patients with major depressive disorder unresponsive to antidepressant treatment: the VAST-D randomized clinical trial. JAMA 2017;318(2):132–45.

158. Sharma V, Smith A, Mazmanian D. Olanzapine in the prevention of postpartum psychosis and mood episodes in bipolar disorder. Bipolar Disord 2006;8(4):400–4.

159. Baastrup PC, Schou M. Lithium as a prophylactic agents. Its effect against recurrent depressions and manic-depressive psychosis. Arch Gen Psychiatry 1967;16(2):162–72.

160. Rush AJ, Trivedi MH, Wisniewski SR, et al. Acute and longer-term outcomes in depressed outpatients requiring one or several treatment steps: a STAR*D report. Am J Psychiatry 2006;163(11):1905–17.

161. Bergink V, Burgerhout KM, Koorengevel KM, et al. Treatment of psychosis and mania in the postpartum period. Am J Psychiatry 2015;172(2):115–23.

162. Bergink V, Bouvy PF, Vervoort JS, et al. Prevention of postpartum psychosis and mania in women at high risk. Am J Psychiatry 2012;169(6):609–15.

163. Austin MP. Puerperal affective psychosis: is there a case for lithium prophylaxis? Br J Psychiatry 1992;161:692–4.

164. Cohen LS, Sichel DA, Robertson LM, et al. Postpartum prophylaxis for women with bipolar disorder. Am J Psychiatry 1995;152(11):1641–5.

165. Wisner KL, Hanusa BH, Peindl KS, et al. Prevention of postpartum episodes in women with bipolar disorder. Biol Psychiatry 2004;56(8):592–6.

Complementary Health Practices for Treating Perinatal Depression

Nafisa Reza, MD[a], Kristina M. Deligiannidis, MD[a,b,c],
Elizabeth H. Eustis, MA[d], Cynthia L. Battle, PhD[d,e,f],*

KEYWORDS

- Complementary • Treatment • Nutraceuticals • Physical activity • Yoga
- Depression • Postpartum • Perinatal

KEY POINTS

- This review examines the evidence regarding common complementary health practices, including natural products (omega-3 fatty acids, folate, vitamin D, selenium, zinc, magnesium, B vitamins) and mind-body practices (physical activity interventions, yoga) in reducing perinatal depression.
- Current evidence regarding efficacy, safety, dosing, and duration of complementary health practices remains limited, yet promising data are emerging regarding the potential depression-reducing effect of omega-3 fatty acids, folate, vitamin D, physical activity, and yoga.
- Adequately powered high-quality studies are necessary to determine the role of complementary health practices for treating perinatal depression.

Disclosure Statement: The authors of this article do not have conflicts of interest relevant to the subject of this article. This article was supported by National Institutes of Health Grants 5K23MH097794 (K.M. Deligiannidis), R01HD81868 (C.L. Battle), R01NR014540 (C.L. Battle & Salisbury); R34MH103570 (C.L. Battle & Weinstock). The views expressed in this article are those of the authors and do not necessarily reflect the position of the NIH.
Conflict of Interest: None.

[a] Department of Psychiatry, Zucker Hillside Hospital, Northwell Health, 75-59 263rd Street, Glen Oaks, NY 11004, USA; [b] Departments of Psychiatry and Obstetrics & Gynecology, Zucker School of Medicine at Hofstra/Northwell, 500 Hofstra Boulevard, Hempstead, NY 11549, USA; [c] Feinstein Institute for Medical Research, 300 Community Drive, Manhasset, NY 11030, USA; [d] Department of Psychiatry and Human Behavior, Warren Alpert Medical School of Brown University, 700 Butler Drive, Providence, RI 02903, USA; [e] Butler Hospital, 345 Blackstone Boulevard, Providence, RI 02906, USA; [f] Center for Women's Behavioral Health, Women & Infants Hospital of Rhode Island, 2 Dudley Street, Providence, RI 02905, USA
* Corresponding author. 345 Blackstone Boulevard, Providence, RI 02906.
E-mail address: Cynthia_Battle@brown.edu

INTRODUCTION

Approximately 14% to 23% of women develop depression during pregnancy and up to 16.7% develop depression within 3 months postdelivery.[1] Perinatal depression (PND) is underdiagnosed and few women receive treatment.[2] Untreated PND is associated with functional impairment and adverse health outcomes for mother and child, including obstetric and neonatal complications[3] and a broad negative impact on child development.[4] Maternal suicide is the leading cause of maternal death occurring within 1 year postpartum.[5] Fortunately, safe and effective treatment options exist, including psychotherapy[6] and antidepressants.[7] However, an understanding of complementary health practices (CHPs) is important, because perinatal women may inquire about nonpharmacologic treatments.

CHPs include a diverse range of practices that are developed outside of mainstream Western medicine. Most CHPs fall into two categories: natural products or mind and body practices. Natural products, including herbs, vitamins, minerals, and probiotics, are the most widely used CHP in the United States. Mind and body practices include techniques that are typically administered or taught by a practitioner. Physical activity interventions may also be conceptualized as a form of CHP.

In general, women suffer from disorders, such as depression and anxiety, more often than men, for which CHPs are commonly pursued.[8] Despite growing popularity of CHP, research is limited. In light of their increased use, we reviewed literature on CHPs for PND. We included specific approaches (ie, omega-3 fatty acids [O-3FA], folate, vitamin D, selenium, zinc, magnesium, B vitamins, physical activity, yoga) based on prevalence of use and availability of evidence from randomized controlled trials (RCT) in PND. In the absence of RCT evidence in PND, we included data from nonrandomized trials and studies addressing impact of these approaches on depressive symptoms within nonclinical populations.

NATURAL PRODUCTS
Omega-3 Fatty Acids

O-3FA are one of the most popular CHPs used in the United States. O-3FA are essential polyunsaturated fatty acids with well-established health benefits.[9] Eicosapentaenoic acid (EPA) and docosahexaenoic acid (DHA) are two important O-3FAs. Guidelines recommend pregnant women consume at least 200 mg/d of DHA.[10] The 2015 to 2020 Dietary Guidelines for Americans[11] and the American College of Obstetricians and Gynecologists (ACOG) recommend pregnant or breastfeeding women consume 8 to 12 ounces of seafood weekly, which provides approximately 250 mg/d of EPA and DHA.[12]

Meta-analyses of RCTs suggest antidepressant benefits of O-3FA in mood disorders overall, but there has been heterogeneity in study design, quality of evidence, and results.[13,14] O-3FA have been studied as augmentation to treatment[15] and as depression monotherapy.[16] The American Psychiatric Association recommends patients with a mood disorder consume 1 g/d EPA + DHA.[17]

Studies on the relationship between serum O-3FA levels or dietary seafood intake and PND have yielded mixed results.[18,19] In a large prospective Danish cohort study including more than 54,000 women, those with the lowest quartile of fish intake were at increased risk of antidepressant treatment postpartum.[20] Several RCTs assessing O-3FA supplementation in the treatment or prevention of PND have not demonstrated benefit.[21] A large double-blind RCT including 2,399 nondepressed pregnant women who received either 800 mg/d DHA plus 100 mg/d EPA or vegetable oil during the last half of pregnancy[22] showed no between-group difference in PND symptoms as measured by the Edinburgh Postnatal Depression Scale (EPDS).[22]

Three double-blind placebo-controlled RCTs in depressed pregnant women found a significant benefit of O-3FA as monotherapy for antenatal depression.[23–25] Another trial, however, did not find any benefit compared with placebo in pregnant women at high risk for PND.[26] A recent systematic review and meta-analysis of 12 studies noted lower levels of EPA and DHA were associated with PND.[19] Given some positive findings from RCTs and meta-analyses in depression and PND, we recommend depressed perinatal women consume 1 g/d EPA + DHA in addition to psychotherapy or pharmacotherapy as recommended by their behavioral health clinician. Further high-quality studies are needed to determine optimal dose and treatment duration. Please see **Table 1** for a summary of research on natural products.

Folate

Folate exists in several forms, including folic acid, folinic acid, and the biologically active 5-methyltetrahydrofolate and participates in the production of nucleic acids and amino acid metabolism. Folate is converted to L-methylfolate, a biologically active form. Folic acid and folinic acid are synthetic forms of dietary folate and require methylenetetrahydrofolate reductase (MTHFR) to be converted into biologically active forms. Polymorphism of MTHFR is common in depressed patients, resulting in impaired transformation of folate to L-methylfolate. Pregnant women and women with the potential for pregnancy are recommended to consume 0.4 to 0.8 mg of folic acid daily.[27] Women at elevated risk for delivering an infant with a neural tube defect are advised to consume 4 mg/d folic acid before and during pregnancy.[27,28]

Studies report an association between low folate and an increased risk of depression.[29] Synthetic forms of dietary folate and L-methylfolate have been tested as adjunctive treatment in depression,[30] but results are inconsistent.[31] No published trials have examined the efficacy of folate monotherapy or augmentation therapy for PND.[32] Epidemiologic data generally do not demonstrate that higher folate intake during pregnancy mitigates PND[33]; however, in one study of 709 pregnant women,[34] lower plasma folate status was associated with antenatal depression. A prospective study of 6,809 women reported that antenatal folic acid supplementation protected against PND; this was especially evident in those with the MTHFR C677T genotype.[35] Another study of 1,592 women found that 6 months of folate supplementation was associated with lower rates of PND.[36]

In summary, in perinatal women with low serum folate levels, folic or folinic acid supplementation carries little risk and may reduce PND risk. However, given lack of clear evidence, it is premature to conclude that doses higher than that recommended by ACOG are effective in PND treatment.

Vitamin D

Vitamin D is a fat-soluble vitamin available as a biologically inert dietary supplement and produced endogenously by the skin after sunlight exposure.[37] 25-hydroxyvitamin D (25-(OH)-D) is the product of the first hydroxylation of vitamin D. The US Recommended Dietary Allowance (RDA) for vitamin D intake during pregnancy and during lactation is 600 IU/d (15 μg). Prenatal vitamins generally contain 400 IU but greater supplemental doses of 1500 to 2000 IU/d of vitamin D may be needed to obtain serum concentrations greater than 30 ng/mL.[38]

Data support a lower risk of subsequent depression with higher serum levels, between 50 and 85 nmol/L.[39] A meta-analysis of observational studies involving 31,424 nonpregnant adults reported low vitamin D levels associated with clinical depression.[40] Recent RCTs report conflicting results.[41] One meta-analysis found an effect size for vitamin D comparable with that of antidepressants,[42] but other meta-analyses did not find a significant reduction in depression in nondeficient patients.[43]

Many studies report lower maternal 25(OH)-D levels to be associated with PND.[37,44] Observational studies identify an association between higher dietary vitamin D intake and a lower prevalence of PND symptoms.[45,46] In contrast, another study including 875 unaffected and 605 women with PND reported serum levels above sufficiency were associated with an increased risk of PND.[47]

To date, only one RCT has assessed efficacy of vitamin D as a treatment of PND. That study reported that 2000 IU/d for at least 8 weeks starting at the onset of the third trimester was associated with reduced depression in late gestation and 8 weeks postpartum, compared with placebo plus typical prenatal vitamins.[48] This study's generalizability is unclear because women with moderate-severe depressive symptoms (ie, EPDS >13) were excluded and nearly 70% of the women were vitamin D deficient.

Vitamin D deficiency should be promptly treated to reduce maternal, fetal, and neonatal health risks associated with deficiency. Treatment of vitamin D deficiency may lower the risk of PND. Larger trials need to be conducted before routine use of vitamin D is recommended for use in nondeficient pregnant women at risk for developing PND.

OTHER NUTRACEUTICALS, MICRONUTRIENTS
Selenium

Selenium is an essential trace element present in many foods like seafood, meat, and breads. The RDA of selenium is 60 μg in pregnancy.[49] Low selenium intake is associated with increased risk for depression.[50] Outcomes of intervention trials have been mixed.[51,52] One RCT investigated selenium supplementation for the prevention of PND.[53] This double blind, placebo-controlled study enrolled 166 healthy first-trimester women. Women received either placebo or 100 μg/d selenium yeast for 6 months until delivery. The mean postpartum EPDS score in the selenium group was lower than that of the control group but the result was not statistically significant.[54]

A large naturalistic prospective study of 475 pregnant women investigated the relationship between risk for PND symptoms and use of several micronutrient supplements, including B vitamins, vitamin D, iron, magnesium, selenium, zinc, and O-3FA.[55] Only selenium use greater than RDA levels reduced the odds of scoring as probable minor depression on the EPDS.

Currently, there is insufficient evidence to conclude that prenatal selenium supplementation prevents or treats PND. High-quality controlled clinical trials should be conducted to determine if selenium supplementation could have a role in the prevention or treatment of PND.

Zinc

Zinc is an essential element required as a cofactor of many enzymes; it is found in red meat, poultry, and beans. The RDA during pregnancy is 11 mg[56] and pregnant women should not take more than 40 mg/d. Studies have reported lower serum zinc concentrations associated with depression,[57] including PND.[58] Several trials have investigated zinc as an adjunct to antidepressants.[59]

Few studies to date have focused on perinatal women and current results are mixed.[55,60] A recent RCT evaluated the effects of zinc sulfate versus magnesium sulfate supplementation versus placebo in preventing PND symptoms and anxiety.[61] This study included 99 healthy early postpartum women. Both supplements were tolerated, but no significant difference in symptoms was found 8 weeks postpartum.

Well-designed placebo-controlled RCTs with zinc in PND are limited. Zinc has potential benefit regarding mood but can interact with medications including antibiotics.[62] At this time zinc cannot be recommended to prevent or treat PND.

Magnesium

Magnesium is a trace mineral that activates many enzymes. The RDA in pregnancy ranges from 360 mg to 400 mg.[63] No clear association between magnesium deficiency and depression has been reported.[64] Few studies to date have focused on perinatal women and current results are mixed as reviewed previously.[55,61] At this time, there is insufficient evidence supporting perinatal magnesium supplementation to treat depression, particularly given the potential interactions with other medications.

B Vitamins

B vitamins function as important coenzymes or the precursors needed to make coenzymes, for metabolic processes. The RDA of riboflavin (B$_2$) during pregnancy is 1.4 mg. The RDA of pyridoxine (B$_6$) in pregnancy is 1.9 mg; pregnant women should not take more than 80 mg/d.[65] The RDA of cobalamin (B$_{12}$) during pregnancy is 2.6 μg.[66]

A few studies support an inverse relationship between riboflavin (B$_2$) intake and depressive symptoms[67]; however, sparse research exists with perinatal women. A prospective cohort study using self-reported dietary intake in 865 pregnant women suggested that consuming food with high riboflavin content was associated with a decreased PND risk.[68]

Deficiency in pyridoxine (vitamin B$_6$) and cobalamin (vitamin B$_{12}$) is associated with increased homocysteine, a proinflammatory amino acid. Studies investigating the association between pyridoxine and depression report inconsistent findings.[69,70] Cobalamin deficiency has been associated with non-PND[71]; however, no clear association has been documented between cobalamin and PND.[32] A few studies have reported a lack of correlation between perinatal plasma cobalamin levels or intake and PND.[34,68] A large study of 905 women with postpartum depression symptoms and 1,951 without symptoms similarly did not find any relationship between depressive symptoms and dietary intake of folate, cobalamin, or pyridoxine at 6 months or 1 year postpartum.[72] Overall, there is insufficient evidence to recommend riboflavin, pyridoxine, or cobalamin supplementation for PND.

MIND AND BODY PRACTICES
Physical Activity

Regular physical activity is an important part of maintaining health and a sense of well-being. A growing literature documents mental health benefits of exercise including increased activity as a strategy for lowering depression. Behavioral, psychological, and physiologic mechanisms have been proposed to explain the mood-enhancing effect of exercise. In contrast to older recommendations to minimize perinatal exercise, ACOG currently endorses regular physical activity (ie, 20–30 minutes daily of moderate intensity activity) among healthy pregnant and postpartum women, and observational studies document numerous benefits of perinatal exercise. In light of potential benefits to overall health and mood, tailored exercise programs have been suggested as promising strategies for improving maternal perinatal mood.

Table 1
Natural products as treatments for perinatal depression: current evidence and recommendations

Natural Product	Recommendation for Use During Pregnancy and Postpartum
Omega-3 fatty acids	• Evidence suggests daily EPA + DHA is well tolerated and may help reduce depression during perinatal period • Consistent with APA guidelines, a daily dose of 1 g/d of EPA + DHA is recommended to help reduce depression, as an adjunct to standard mental health treatment
Folate	• Modest support currently exists for an antidepressant effect of folate augmentation in nonperinatal populations, with little evidence of risk • ACOG recommends 600 μg of folate daily to reduce risk of neural tube defects. Adhering to this dose is important for fetal health and may also help reduce maternal depression, particularly in women with low serum folate levels
S-adenosyl-L-methionine	• No RCTs to date with depressed pregnant women; only one study has examined S-adenosyl-L-methionine for postpartum depressive symptoms • Currently not enough evidence regarding efficacy and safety to recommend S-adenosyl-L-methionine for perinatal depression
Vitamin D	• Only one RCT has examined vitamin D as a treatment of perinatal depression • Treating vitamin D deficiency is critical for maternal-child health; however, there is currently insufficient evidence to recommend vitamin D for perinatal depression in nondeficient women
Selenium	• No RCTs have evaluated selenium as a treatment of perinatal depression; one RCT has examined preventative effect • Currently not enough evidence regarding efficacy to recommend selenium as a treatment of perinatal depression.
Zinc	• No RCTs have evaluated zinc as a treatment of perinatal depression; one RCT examined preventative effect • Currently not enough evidence regarding efficacy to recommend zinc as a treatment of perinatal depression
Magnesium	• No RCTs have evaluated magnesium as a treatment of perinatal depression; one RCT examined preventative effect • Currently not enough evidence regarding efficacy to recommend zinc as a treatment of perinatal depression
B vitamins	• No RCTs have evaluated B vitamins as treatments of perinatal depression • Currently not enough evidence regarding efficacy to recommend riboflavin, pyridoxine, or cobalamin for perinatal depression

Although exercise has been tested as an intervention for depression in numerous studies in the general population, only a few trials have examined the effects of exercise among depressed perinatal women. Six RCTs have examined various forms of exercise for postpartum women with depression symptoms, and one open trial has examined an exercise intervention for depressed pregnant women.

Among the RCTs examining exercise for PND, the type of exercise intervention has varied, including group-based pram-walking,[73] facility-based group exercise,[74] and individualized exercise interventions tailored to participant needs and preferences.[75,76] The amount of physical activity promoted by these programs and duration has also varied, yet all involved mild-moderate intensity levels of activity and exertion. With one exception,[73] comparison conditions have involved no-treatment control groups. Findings regarding efficacy are generally encouraging, yet not all studies yielded positive findings. Two RCTs[73,74] found the exercise group experienced greater depression reductions than the control group; this includes a small trial (N = 19) that found that a twice-weekly pram-walking intervention was more effective than weekly social support for improving mood, and a larger study (N = 80) that found greater symptom reduction among women who participated in a group/individual exercise program versus standard care. In a later trial with 94 postpartum women, Daley and colleagues[76] documented greater depression reduction in an exercise group; however, differences were small and not maintained at 12-month follow-up. Da Costa and colleagues[75] reported no differences between exercise and control groups, yet additional analyses revealed that women with high baseline depression scores did experience significant depression reductions compared with women with high scores assigned to the control condition. Finally, two other RCTs[77,78] did not find an effect of group assignment on depression outcomes, one[77] noting that problems with adherence to the exercise intervention may have accounted for lack of effect.

In terms of prenatal interventions, only one small study has examined an exercise program for pregnant women with depression. In a nonrandomized trial with second- and third-trimester pregnant women, Battle and Abrantes[79] found clinically significant depression reductions and increases in physical activity following a 10-week lifestyle physical activity intervention. This intervention is currently being tested in a larger RCT (NCT02474862; clinicaltrials.gov).

Research on physical activity as a treatment of PND is new, and studies to date have been limited by small samples and lack of comparison groups that control for time, attention, and other concurrent depression treatment. Moreover, few trials have used objective physical activity measurement (eg, accelerometry, the gold standard in exercise research). Still, current evidence suggests that physical activity approaches are viewed as acceptable by perinatal women and providers, and no safety concerns have been documented. ACOG already recommends regular moderate-intensity physical activity among perinatal women and suggests that prenatal care providers should actively encourage their depressed patients without medical contraindications to adhere to these guidelines, because regular exercise may promote better mental and obstetric health. Providers should regularly assess patients' activity over the perinatal period to gauge ongoing safety and difficulties overcoming barriers to activity. Given the strong evidence for acceptability and potential for improving maternal health and mood, additional high-quality studies are needed to establish whether exercise interventions are efficacious as a treatment of PND, to clarify the optimal dose of exercise, and examine effective strategies for promoting adherence. Please see **Table 2** for a summary of research on physical activity and yoga interventions.

Yoga

Yoga is an ancient practice that varies in style, yet typically combines three components: (1) physical postures, (2) breath control, and (3) meditation. A growing proportion of the United States and Canadian population practices yoga, and its popularity is higher among women than men. In recent decades the impact of yoga on physical and mental health has been examined (eg, to improve cardiovascular health, reduce pain). In light of putative mechanisms by which yoga could improve depression, yoga has been tested as a potential intervention for depression in the general population. This literature suggests that yoga is more effective in treating depression than placebo and comparable with aerobic exercise and antidepressant medication, despite methodologic limitations in studies to date.

Recently, prenatal and postpartum yoga have been studied as potential interventions to treat depression. Depressed pregnant women have found prenatal yoga to be acceptable, feasible, and safe.[80–82] In terms of open trials, one study examined a yoga program for depressed pregnant women and found significant decreases in depression via self-report and observer-rated measures.[80] Another trial reported significant reductions in depressive symptoms following a yoga program in a mixed patient sample with a range of symptoms.[83] RCTs of yoga for PND have compared brief yoga (or yoga/tai chi) programs with a range of conditions including waitlist,[84] massage and treatment as usual,[85] social support,[86] and parenting education,[87] reporting greater reductions in depressive symptoms in yoga versus waitlist, treatment as usual, and parenting education, and similar reductions versus massage and social support. These studies were conducted with diverse samples. Some studies were limited by use of a less typical style of yoga (eg, brief sessions with postures only), or reliance on self-report measures. Other RCTs have compared yoga programs with treatment as usual in depressed and/or anxious women[82] and a perinatal health education condition in depressed women,[81] and have reported decreases in depression, yet with minimal or no significant differences versus comparison conditions. One RCT examined a postpartum yoga intervention versus waitlist for women with depression up to 12 months postpartum and found that participants in the yoga condition reported greater improvements in depression.[88]

Although more research is needed, the existing body of research on prenatal and postpartum yoga is encouraging in terms of feasibility, acceptability, preliminary efficacy, and patient safety. Perinatal women without medical contraindications or activity restrictions may experience some mood benefit from a regular yoga practice tailored for perinatal women. The appropriateness of a yoga program should be assessed across the perinatal period, because medical status and activity restrictions may change. Rigorous, fully powered RCTs are needed to examine the efficacy of yoga for depressed women during pregnancy and postpartum, and explore questions of the adequate "dose" of yoga, and safety considerations. Future research should evaluate yoga interventions that are consistent with typical prenatal yoga classes offered in community settings, to maximize generalizability, and should use observer-rated measures of depression outcomes, in addition to self-report measures.

SUMMARY

Given high levels of interest in CHPs during the perinatal period, there is a need for research addressing acceptability, safety, and efficacy of these interventions. Large-scale surveys suggest many perinatal women already seek out CHP for potential health benefits, even in the absence of clear safety and efficacy data, and a substantial subset of perinatal women report that their prenatal care providers do not ask about their use of CHPs.[89] As such, it is important for providers to routinely inquire about patients' interest in and use of CHPs, and additional research is needed to provide clear data to guide decisions about which products and practices are helpful and safe.

With a vast array of CHPs, we did not attempt to review evidence for all products or interventions. We examined data regarding some of the most commonly used CHPs, including various natural products and vitamins and popular mind and body approaches. Until subsequent research is conducted and questions answered, our review has found encouraging preliminary evidence supporting efficacy of O-3FA, folate, vitamin D (in cases of deficiency), physical activity interventions, and prenatal/postpartum yoga for reducing or preventing PND symptoms. However, some approaches have only been examined during pregnancy, and others only in the postpartum. At this time there is insufficient evidence for the efficacy of selenium,

Table 2
Physical activity and yoga as treatments for perinatal depression: current evidence and recommendations

Mind or Body Intervention	Recommendation for Use During Pregnancy and Postpartum
Physical activity	• Some evidence exists suggesting exercise may be efficacious in lowering postpartum depression without adverse effect; less evidence for antenatal depression, but positive results documented in one open trial. • ACOG recommends moderate-intensity physical activity for 20–30 minutes on most days for pregnant women with uncomplicated pregnancies, and resuming (or starting) exercise when medically cleared postpartum. • In addition to health benefits, following ACOG exercise guidelines may serve as an effective adjunct to standard mental health treatment to help improve mood among women with perinatal depression. • Because of difficulty adhering to exercise programs while pregnant or postpartum, we recommend providers actively support women in increasing activity over the perinatal period to adhere to ACOG guidelines and obtain potential health and mood benefits.
Yoga	• Some evidence exists suggesting prenatal and postpartum yoga may be efficacious in lowering perinatal depression. • Modified yoga is an activity recommended as "safe" by ACOG for women engaging in regular physical activity during pregnancy; guidelines note that "hot yoga" and postures that result in decreased venous return and hypotension should be avoided. No safety concerns have been documented with yoga interventions studied to date with perinatal women. • A modified yoga practice is one strategy for adhering to ACOG physical activity guidelines, and preliminary evidence suggests that prenatal and postpartum yoga may also serve as an efficacious adjunctive intervention to help improve mood among women with perinatal depression.

zinc, magnesium, and B vitamins. Given their acceptability and availability, CHPs are an important area for future study to determine their utility as either adjunctive interventions or monotherapy to reduce PND.

ACKNOWLEDGMENTS

The authors acknowledge Janice Lester, MLS, Reference and Education Librarian, Health Science Library, Long Island Jewish Medical Center, Northwell Health.

REFERENCES

1. Gaynes BN, Gavin N, Meltzer-Brody S, et al. Perinatal depression: prevalence, screening accuracy, and screening outcomes. Evid Rep Technol Assess (Summ) 2005;(119):1–8.
2. Cox EQ, Sowa NA, Meltzer-Brody SE, et al. The perinatal depression treatment cascade: baby steps toward improving outcomes. J Clin Psychiatry 2016; 77(9):1189–200.
3. Grote NK, Bridge JA, Gavin AR, et al. A meta-analysis of depression during pregnancy and the risk of preterm birth, low birth weight, and intrauterine growth restriction. Arch Gen Psychiatry 2010;67(10):1012–24.
4. Britton JR. Infant temperament and maternal anxiety and depressed mood in the early postpartum period. Women Health 2011;51(1):55–71.

5. Knight M, Nair M, Tuffnell D, et al. Saving lives, improving mothers' care: surveillance of maternal deaths in the UK 2012-14 and lessons learned to inform maternity care from the UK and Ireland confidential enquiries into maternal deaths and morbidity 2009-2014. Oxford (UK): National Perinatal Epidemiology Unit, University of Oxford, UK; 2016.

6. Milgrom J, Gemmill AW, Ericksen J, et al. Treatment of postnatal depression with cognitive behavioural therapy, sertraline and combination therapy: a randomised controlled trial. Aust N Z J Psychiatry 2015;49(3):236–45.

7. Wisner KL, Hanusa BH, Perel JM, et al. Postpartum depression: a randomized trial of sertraline versus nortriptyline. J Clin Psychopharmacol 2006;26(4):353–60.

8. Wu P, Fuller C, Liu X, et al. Use of complementary and alternative medicine among women with depression: results of a national survey. Psychiatr Serv 2007;58(3):349–56.

9. Emmett PM, Jones LR, Golding J. Pregnancy diet and associated outcomes in the Avon longitudinal study of parents and children. Nutr Rev 2015;73(Suppl 3):154–74.

10. Koletzko B, Lien E, Agostoni C, et al. The roles of long-chain polyunsaturated fatty acids in pregnancy, lactation and infancy: review of current knowledge and consensus recommendations. J Perinat Med 2008;36(1):5–14.

11. U.S. Department of Health and Human Services, U.S. Department of Agriculture. 2015–2020 dietary guidelines for Americans. 8th edition. Washington, DC; 2015. Available at: https://health.gov/dietaryguidelines/2015/guidelines/table-of-contents/.

12. American College of Obstetricians and Gynecologists. Nutrition During Pregnancy. Washington, DC: American College of Obstetricians and Gynecologists; 2010. Available at: https://www.acog.org/-/media/Womens-Health/nutrition-in-pregnancy.pdf.

13. Appleton KM, Sallis HM, Perry R, et al. Omega-3 fatty acids for depression in adults. Cochrane Database Syst Rev 2015;(11):CD004692.

14. Mocking RJ, Harmsen I, Assies J, et al. Meta-analysis and meta-regression of omega-3 polyunsaturated fatty acid supplementation for major depressive disorder. Transl Psychiatry 2016;6:e756.

15. Browne JC, Scott KM, Silvers KM. Fish consumption in pregnancy and omega-3 status after birth are not associated with postnatal depression. J Affect Disord 2006;90(2–3):131–9.

16. Kumar R, Robson KM. A prospective study of emotional disorders in childbearing women. Br J Psychiatry 1984;144:35–47.

17. Freeman MP, Fava M, Lake J, et al. Complementary and alternative medicine in major depressive disorder: the American Psychiatric Association Task Force report. J Clin Psychiatry 2010;71(6):669–81.

18. Newberry S, Chung M, Booth M, et al. Omega-3 fatty acids and maternal and child health: an updated systematic review. Rockville (MD): Agency for Healthcare Research and Quality (US); 2016.

19. Lin PY, Chang CH, Chong MF, et al. Polyunsaturated fatty acids in perinatal depression: a systematic review and meta-analysis. Biol Psychiatry 2017;82(8):560–9.

20. Strom M, Mortensen EL, Halldorsson TI, et al. Fish and long-chain n-3 polyunsaturated fatty acid intakes during pregnancy and risk of postpartum depression: a prospective study based on a large national birth cohort. Am J Clin Nutr 2009; 90(1):149–55.

21. Freeman MP, Davis M, Sinha P, et al. Omega-3 fatty acids and supportive psychotherapy for perinatal depression: a randomized placebo-controlled study. J Affect Disord 2008;110(1–2):142–8.

22. Makrides M, Gibson RA, McPhee AJ, et al. Effect of DHA supplementation during pregnancy on maternal depression and neurodevelopment of young children a randomized controlled trial. JAMA 2010;304(15):1675–83.

23. Su KP, Huang SY, Chiu TH, et al. Omega-3 fatty acids for major depressive disorder during pregnancy: results from a randomized, double-blind, placebo-controlled trial. J Clin Psychiatry 2008;69(4):644–51.

24. Kaviani M, Saniee L, Azima S, et al. The effect of omega-3 fatty acid supplementation on maternal depression during pregnancy: a double blind randomized controlled clinical trial. Int J Community Based Nurs Midwifery 2014;2(3):142–7.

25. Farshbaf-Khalili A, Mohammad-Alizadeh S, Farshbaf-Khalili A, et al. Fish-oil supplementation and maternal mental health: A triple-blind, randomized controlled trial. Iranian Red Crescent Medical Journal 2017;19(1):e36237.

26. Vaz JD, Farias DR, Adegboye ARA, et al. Omega-3 supplementation from pregnancy to postpartum to prevent depressive symptoms: a randomized placebo-controlled trial. BMC Pregnancy Childbirth 2017;17(1):180.

27. Force USPST, Bibbins-Domingo K, Grossman DC, et al. Folic acid supplementation for the prevention of neural tube defects: US Preventive Services Task Force recommendation statement. JAMA 2017;317(2):183–9.

28. Wilson RD, Genetics C, Wilson RD, et al. Pre-conception folic acid and multivitamin supplementation for the primary and secondary prevention of neural tube defects and other folic acid-sensitive congenital anomalies. J Obstet Gynaecol Can 2015;37(6):534–52.

29. Beydoun MA, Shroff MR, Beydoun HA, et al. Serum folate, vitamin B-12, and homocysteine and their association with depressive symptoms among U.S. adults. Psychosom Med 2010;72(9):862–73.

30. Papakostas GI, Shelton RC, Zajecka JM, et al. L-methylfolate as adjunctive therapy for SSRI-resistant major depression: results of two randomized, double-blind, parallel-sequential trials. Am J Psychiatry 2012;169(12):1267–74.

31. Taylor MJ, Carney S, Geddes J, et al. Folate for depressive disorders. Cochrane Database Syst Rev 2003;(2):CD003390.

32. Sparling TM, Henschke N, Nesbitt RC, et al. The role of diet and nutritional supplementation in perinatal depression: a systematic review. Matern Child Nutr 2017;13(1). https://doi.org/10.1111/mcn.12235.

33. Cho YJ, Han JY, Choi JS, et al. Prenatal multivitamins containing folic acid do not decrease prevalence of depression among pregnant women. J Obstet Gynaecol 2008;28(5):482–4.

34. Chong MFF, Wong JXY, Colega M, et al. Relationships of maternal folate and vitamin B12 status during pregnancy with perinatal depression: the GUSTO study. J Psychiatr Res 2014;55:110–6.

35. Lewis SJ, Araya R, Leary S, et al. Folic acid supplementation during pregnancy may protect against depression 21 months after pregnancy, an effect modified by MTHFR C677T genotype. Eur J Clin Nutr 2012;66(1):97–103.

36. Yan J, Liu Y, Cao L, et al. Association between duration of folic acid supplementation during pregnancy and risk of postpartum depression. Nutrients 2017;9(11) [pii:E1206].

37. Williams JA, Romero VC, Clinton CM, et al. Vitamin D levels and perinatal depressive symptoms in women at risk: a secondary analysis of the mothers, omega-3, and mental health study. BMC Pregnancy Childbirth 2016;16(1):203.

38. Holick MF, Binkley NC, Bischoff-Ferrari HA, et al. Evaluation, treatment, and prevention of vitamin D deficiency: an endocrine society clinical practice guideline. J Clin Endocrinol Metab 2011;96(7):1911–30.

39. Maddock J, Berry DJ, Geoffroy MC, et al. Vitamin D and common mental disorders in mid-life: cross-sectional and prospective findings. Clin Nutr 2013;32(5): 758–64.

40. Anglin RE, Samaan Z, Walter SD, et al. Vitamin D deficiency and depression in adults: systematic review and meta-analysis. Br J Psychiatry 2013;202:100–7.

41. Rejnmark L, Bislev LS, Cashman KD, et al. Non-skeletal health effects of vitamin D supplementation: a systematic review on findings from meta-analyses summarizing trial data. PLoS One 2017;12(7):e0180512.

42. Spedding S. Vitamin D and depression: a systematic review and meta-analysis comparing studies with and without biological flaws. Nutrients 2014;6(4): 1501–18.

43. Gowda U, Mutowo MP, Smith BJ, et al. Vitamin D supplementation to reduce depression in adults: meta-analysis of randomized controlled trials. Nutrition 2015;31(3):421–9.

44. Gur EB, Gokduman A, Turan GA, et al. Mid-pregnancy vitamin D levels and postpartum depression. Eur J Obstet Gynecol Reprod Biol 2014;179:110–6.

45. Miyake Y, Tanaka K, Okubo H, et al. Dietary vitamin D intake and prevalence of depressive symptoms during pregnancy in Japan. Nutrition 2015;31(1):160–5.

46. Brandenbarg J, Vrijkotte TGM, Goedhart G, et al. Maternal early-pregnancy vitamin D status is associated with maternal depressive symptoms in the Amsterdam born children and their development cohort. Psychosom Med 2012;74(7): 751–7.

47. Nielsen NO, Strom M, Boyd HA, et al. Vitamin D status during pregnancy and the risk of subsequent postpartum depression: a case-control study. PLoS One 2013; 8(11):e80686.

48. Vaziri F, Nasiri S, Tavana Z, et al. A randomized controlled trial of vitamin D supplementation on perinatal depression: in Iranian pregnant mothers. BMC Pregnancy Childbirth 2016;16:239.

49. Institute of Medicine (US) Panel on Dietary Antioxidants and Related Compounds. Dietary reference intakes for vitamin C, vitamin E, selenium, and carotenoids. Washington, DC: National Academies Press (US); 2000. Copyright 2000 by the National Academy of Sciences. All rights reserved.

50. Pasco JA, Jacka FN, Williams LJ, et al. Dietary selenium and major depression: a nested case-control study. Complement Ther Med 2012;20(3):119–23.

51. Benton D, Cook R. The impact of selenium supplementation on mood. Biol Psychiatry 1991;29(11):1092–8.

52. Rayman M, Thompson A, Warren-Perry M, et al. Impact of selenium on mood and quality of life: a randomized, controlled trial. Biol Psychiatry 2006;59(2):147–54.

53. Mokhber N, Namjoo M, Tara F, et al. Effect of supplementation with selenium on postpartum depression: a randomized double-blind placebo-controlled trial. J Matern Fetal Neonatal Med 2011;24(1):104–8.

54. Miller BJ, Murray L, Beckmann MM, et al. Dietary supplements for preventing postnatal depression. Cochrane Database Syst Rev 2013;(10):CD009104.

55. Leung BM, Kaplan BJ, Field CJ, et al. Prenatal micronutrient supplementation and postpartum depressive symptoms in a pregnancy cohort. BMC Pregnancy Childbirth 2013;13:2.

56. Institute of Medicine (US) Panel on Micronutrients. Dietary Reference Intakes for Vitamin A, Vitamin K, Arsenic, Boron, Chromium, Copper, Iodine, Iron, Manganese, Molybdenum, Nickel, Silicon, Vanadium, and Zinc. Washington (DC): National Academies Press (US); 2001. https://doi.org/10.17226/10026. Available from: https://www.ncbi.nlm.nih.gov/books/NBK222310/.

57. Lai J, Moxey A, Nowak G, et al. The efficacy of zinc supplementation in depression: systematic review of randomised controlled trials. J Affect Disord 2012; 136(1–2):e31–9.
58. Roomruangwong C, Kanchanatawan B, Sirivichayakul S, et al. Strongly predict prenatal depression and physio-somatic symptoms, which all together predict postnatal depressive symptoms. Mol Neurobiol 2017;54(2):1500–12.
59. Siwek M, Dudek D, Paul IA, et al. Zinc supplementation augments efficacy of imipramine in treatment resistant patients: a double blind, placebo-controlled study. J Affect Disord 2009;118(1–3):187–95.
60. Wojcik J, Dudek D, Schlegel-Zawadzka M, et al. Antepartum/postpartum depressive symptoms and serum zinc and magnesium levels. Pharmacol Rep 2006; 58(4):571–6.
61. Fard FE, Mirghafourvand M, Mohammad-Alizadeh Charandabi S, et al. Effects of zinc and magnesium supplements on postpartum depression and anxiety: a randomized controlled clinical trial. Women Health 2017;57(9):1115–28.
62. Lomaestro BM, Bailie GR. Absorption interactions with fluoroquinolones. 1995 update. Drug Saf 1995;12(5):314–33.
63. Institute of Medicine. Dietary reference intakes for calcium, phosphorus, magnesium, vitamin D, and fluoride. Washington, DC: National Academies Press; 1997.
64. Derom ML, Sayon-Orea C, Martinez-Ortega JM, et al. Magnesium and depression: a systematic review. Nutr Neurosci 2013;16(5):191–206.
65. Institute of Medicine (US). Standing committee on the scientific evaluation of dietary reference intakes and its panel on folate, Other B vitamins, and choline. Dietary reference intakes for thiamin, riboflavin, niacin, vitamin B6, folate, vitamin B12, pantothenic acid, biotin, and choline. Washington (DC): National Academies Press (US); 1998. https://doi.org/10.17226/6015. Available at: https://www.ncbi.nlm.nih.gov/books/NBK114310/.
66. Kaiser L, Allen LH, American Dietetic Association. Position of the American Dietetic Association: nutrition and lifestyle for a healthy pregnancy outcome. J Am Diet Assoc 2008;108(3):553–61.
67. Murakami K, Miyake Y, Sasaki S, et al. Dietary folate, riboflavin, vitamin B-6, and vitamin B-12 and depressive symptoms in early adolescence: the Ryukyus Child Health Study. Psychosom Med 2010;72(8):763–8.
68. Miyake Y, Sasaki S, Tanaka K, et al. Dietary folate and vitamins B12, B6, and B2 intake and the risk of postpartum depression in Japan: the Osaka Maternal and Child Health Study. J Affect Disord 2006;96(1–2):133–8.
69. Hvas AM, Juul S, Bech P, et al. Vitamin B6 level is associated with symptoms of depression. Psychother Psychosom 2004;73(6):340–3.
70. Ford AH, Flicker L, Thomas J, et al. Vitamins B12, B6, and folic acid for onset of depressive symptoms in older men: results from a 2-year placebo-controlled randomized trial. J Clin Psychiatry 2008;69(8):1203–9.
71. Mikkelsen K, Stojanovska L, Prakash M, et al. The effects of vitamin B on the immune/cytokine network and their involvement in depression. Maturitas 2017;96:58–71.
72. Blunden CH, Inskip HM, Robinson SM, et al. Postpartum depressive symptoms: the B-vitamin link. Ment Health Fam Med 2012;9(1):5–13.
73. Armstrong K, Edwards H. The effectiveness of a pram-walking exercise programme in reducing depressive symptomatology for postnatal women. Int J Nurs Pract 2004;10(4):177–94.
74. Heh SS, Huang LH, Ho SM, et al. Effectiveness of an exercise support program in reducing the severity of postnatal depression in Taiwanese women. Birth 2008; 35(1):60–5.

75. DaCosta D, Lowensteyn I, Abrahamowicz M, et al. A randomized clinical trial of exercise to alleviate postpartum depressed mood. J Psychosom Obstet Gynaecol 2009;30(3):191–200.

76. Daley AJ, Blamey RV, Jolly K, et al. A pragmatic randomized controlled trial to evaluate the effectiveness of a facilitated exercise intervention as a treatment for postnatal depression: the PAM-PeRS trial. Psychol Med 2015;45(11):2413–25.

77. Forsyth J, Boath E, Henshaw C, et al. Exercise as an adjunct treatment for postpartum depression for women living in an inner city: a pilot study. Health Care Women Int 2017;38(6):635–9.

78. Daley A, Winter H, Grimmett C, et al. Feasibility of an exercise intervention for women with postnatal depression: a pilot randomised controlled trial. Br J Gen Pract 2008;58(548):178–83.

79. Battle CL, Abrantes AM. Tailored physical activity interventions as innovative means to address women's perinatal mental health. Swansea (Wales): International Marce Society; 2014.

80. Battle CL, Uebelacker LA, Magee SR, et al. Potential for prenatal yoga to serve as an intervention to treat depression during pregnancy. Womens Health Issues 2015;25(2):134–41.

81. Uebelacker LA, Battle CL, Sutton KA, et al. A pilot randomized controlled trial comparing prenatal yoga to perinatal health education for antenatal depression. Arch Womens Ment Health 2016;19(3):543–7.

82. Davis K, Goodman SH, Leiferman J, et al. A randomized controlled trial of yoga for pregnant women with symptoms of depression and anxiety. Complement Ther Clin Pract 2015;21(3):166–72.

83. Muzik M, Hamilton SE, Lisa Rosenblum K, et al. Mindfulness yoga during pregnancy for psychiatrically at-risk women: preliminary results from a pilot feasibility study. Complement Ther Clin Pract 2012;18(4):235–40.

84. Field T, Diego M, Delgado J, et al. Tai chi/yoga reduces prenatal depression, anxiety and sleep disturbances. Complement Ther Clin Pract 2013;19(1):6–10.

85. Field T, Diego M, Hernandez-Reif M, et al. Yoga and massage therapy reduce prenatal depression and prematurity. J Bodyw Mov Ther 2012;16(2):204–9.

86. Field T, Diego M, Delgado J, et al. Yoga and social support reduce prenatal depression, anxiety and cortisol. J Bodyw Mov Ther 2013;17(4):397–403.

87. Mitchell J, Field T, Diego M, et al. Yoga reduces prenatal depression symptoms. Psychology 2012;3:782–6.

88. Buttner MM, Brock RL, O'Hara MW, et al. Efficacy of yoga for depressed postpartum women: a randomized controlled trial. Complement Ther Clin Pract 2015;21(2):94–100.

89. Hall HR, Jolly K. Women's use of complementary and alternative medicines during pregnancy: a cross-sectional study. Midwifery 2014;30(5):499–505.

Recognizing and Managing Postpartum Psychosis
A Clinical Guide for Obstetric Providers

Lauren M. Osborne, MD

KEYWORDS

- Postpartum psychosis • Bipolar disorder • Perinatal psychiatric disorders
- Treatment

KEY POINTS

- Postpartum psychosis (PPP) is a rare psychiatric emergency that can endanger the lives of the mother and child.
- It most often arises within 10 days of childbirth and is characterized by bizarre thoughts and/or behavior, alterations of consciousness, and mood fluctuation.
- The single biggest risk factor is a personal history of bipolar disorder, and most women with PPP will go on to develop bipolar disorder.
- It carries high rates of suicide and infanticide, and suspected cases require psychiatric evaluation as soon as possible.
- Treatment requires hospitalization and aggressive pharmacologic management.

INTRODUCTION

Postpartum psychosis (PPP) is at once the most dangerous and the least understood of perinatal psychiatric disorders. It affects 1 to 2 per 1000 women and constitutes a true psychiatric emergency, one that requires immediate hospitalization and treatment.[1,2] The lack of knowledge about what it is, how to recognize it, and how to treat it, combined with stigma about perinatal psychiatric disorders in general and the lack of appropriate treatment venues, means that it is often missed, by both obstetricians and psychiatrists, with sometimes tragic consequences.

PPP has been noted since antiquity. Hippocrates described the first case known to the medical literature in 400 BC; his patient was delusional, confused, and had

Dr L.M. Osborne has no commercial or financial conflicts of interest. She receives funding from the Brain and Behavior Foundation (YI 2016 23788) and from the National Institute of Mental Health (1K23 MH110607-01A1).
Departments of Psychiatry & Behavioral Sciences and Gynecology & Obstetrics, Women's Mood Disorders Center, Johns Hopkins University School of Medicine, 550 North Broadway, Suite 305, Baltimore, MD 21205, USA
E-mail address: lmosborne@jhmi.edu

insomnia within 6 days of a twin birth.[3] A medieval gynecologist attributed the disorder to "too much moisture in the womb, causing the brain to fill with water."[4] By the late eighteenth century, German and French obstetricians and neurologists were beginning to write more frequently about the disease. In 1858, French psychiatrist Louis Victor Marcé[5] published his *Treatise on the Madness of Women who are Pregnant, Recently Delivered, or Nursing*.[5] Marcé's carefully observed treatise, although suggesting treatments that today seem woefully barbaric (applying leeches to the vulva, for example), is a model of observation; Marcé saw in his postpartum mothers the same symptoms that doctors struggle to control today. His observations led him to conjecture about the role of the immune response and the endocrine system, 2 systems that today are widely acknowledged to contribute to postpartum mental illness.

CLINICAL PRESENTATION

The name PPP is not, perhaps, the best moniker for an illness that is at least as much an affective, or mood, disorder as it is a psychotic disorder. Many clinicians mistakenly think that the term can be applied to any psychotic symptoms in the postpartum period or that its clinical features will be identical to those of schizophrenia or other primary psychotic disorders. In fact, the symptoms of PPP are distinctive and unique. The onset is typically sudden and occurs within the first 2 weeks post partum.[6-8] The literature has frequently described the distinctive clinical features (**Box 1**), which include a delirium-like waxing and waning of consciousness, disorganization and confusion, depersonalization, and bizarre delusions (often concerning the child or childbirth). Early warning symptoms include insomnia, anxiety, irritability, or mood fluctuation. Although the psychotic symptoms are often the most dramatic manifestation, women also present with mood symptoms: mania (can be irritable or elevated), depressive symptoms, or mixed symptoms. A recent clinical cohort study tracked the phenotypic characteristics of 130 consecutive cases of PPP and used latent class analysis to describe 3 separate symptom profiles:

1. Cases characterized by mania and/or agitation, with irritability much more common than elevated mood (34%)
2. Cases characterized by depression and/or anxiety (41%)
3. Cases showing an atypical or mixed profile (25%)[9]

Across all cases, 25% of patients were disorganized, 20% disoriented, 10% had disturbed consciousness, and 5% developed catatonia. Seventy-two percent had abnormal thought content, which most often consisted of persecutory delusions; a minority had frank hallucinations. See **Boxes 2–4** for representative clinical case presentations.

Box 1
Clinical features of postpartum psychosis

- Disorganization
- Confusion
- Depersonalization
- Insomnia
- Irritability
- Abnormal thought content (delusions and/or hallucinations)
- Abnormal mood (mania or agitation, depression, mixed)

Box 2
Clinical case presentation 1

Postpartum psychosis with manic features

Ms A was a high-achieving professional with no prior psychiatric history who had a twin birth 12 days before her psychiatric presentation. Her babies had been born at term by a planned cesarean delivery because of chorioamnionitis; antibiotic therapy was successful, and she left the hospital on time 4 days after the birth. She slept very little in the hospital and was noted by the nurses to be extremely vigilant about the babies and mildly anxious. Her family reported that she did not sleep at all for 6 days following her hospital discharge. She expressed great anxiety about arrangements at home (worrying about clothes, diapers, and the like) and about the ability of other family members to manage the twins. She was exclusively breastfeeding until 2 days before presentation, when her family dissuaded her from breastfeeding in the hope that she would be able to sleep more; the intervention did not help. On the day of presentation, she began to be suspicious of several family members, accusing them of poisoning the babies' bottles, and began to hide the bottles in secret locations around the house. When her mother suggested that they drive to the hospital, the patient bolted from the car into traffic and was found several hours later by a police officer who drove her to the emergency department. On arrival, the patient was oriented to her name and the date but was unsure where she was, spoke very quickly and was uninterruptable, and talked loudly about the cameras she was sure were watching her in the emergency department and about the physicians, whom she thought were in league with her family to poison the infants.

CAUSE AND RISK FACTORS

PPP is one of the few psychiatric disorders with a clear biological trigger: childbirth. The nineteenth-century psychiatrists who first described it (Esquirol[10], Marcé[5]) noted that symptoms were often associated with pregnancies that had gone awry because of infection, preeclampsia (PE), hypertension, or other medical problems[5]; but more

Box 3
Clinical case presentation 2

Postpartum psychosis with depressed features

Ms B was a sheltered young woman from an insular immigrant community. She had experienced childhood trauma and had a known history of depression and anxiety, successfully treated with antidepressants in the past. She had been well throughout her pregnancy, on no medication; but within 5 days of an uncomplicated spontaneous vaginal birth she became disoriented at home and was unable to find her way from her bedroom to the living room. Over the next several days, her family reported that she moved very slowly and seemed confused; she had a poor appetite, did not seem to understand how to hold or care for the baby, and spent much of the day lying in bed but did not seem able to sleep. She began to make worrisome statements, such as "I'm not here" and "I didn't have a baby." The patient's general practitioner prescribed an antidepressant, which did not help her symptoms; the patient became increasingly confused and unable to complete daily activities, such as showering and eating. The family took over the care of the baby and assigned a family member to care for the patient at home. Several weeks later, the situation had not improved; the family presented to a psychiatrist. The patient was oriented to her name only; she could not name the season or what type of building she was in; she clung to her sister's hand and was unable to find the door of the room she was in. When she was asked about her baby, the patient stated "I don't have a baby, I'm not married."

Box 4
Clinical case presentation 3

Postpartum psychosis with mixed features

Ms C was an elementary school teacher who was quite knowledgeable about mental health. She had no prior psychiatric history but had 2 first-degree relatives with bipolar 1 disorder, one of whom had had multiple hospitalizations and was eventually stabilized on lithium. Her pregnancy was uneventful; but labor lasted more than 36 hours and ended in an emergency cesarean delivery, which the patient found traumatic. Two days after discharge, she represented to the hospital stating she had had a panic attack in the middle of the night and was unable to sleep; this was her first panic attack. The overnight resident deemed her anxious but stable, treated her with lorazepam, and discharged her. She represented several hours later complaining of continued insomnia and anxiety. The consulting psychiatrist could elicit no symptoms of frank mania or psychosis but was concerned about her anxiety, insomnia, and family history of bipolar disorder. Upon discharge she was prescribed lorazepam 3 times daily and was referred to a perinatal psychiatrist who would see her twice weekly. At her second outpatient visit, the patient reported that she was now sleeping 6 hours nightly but continued to feel anxious. The psychiatrist started sertraline at 25 mg. Two days later, the patient's partner called the psychiatrist stating that the patient was writhing on the floor complaining of bugs crawling over her skin and had been agitated and pacing just before. By the time the patient arrived in the emergency department for evaluation, she was mute and catatonic.

---

recent studies have been inconclusive about whether medical factors in pregnancy consistently predict the risk for the disorder, with several studies finding that no pregnancy-related or obstetric factors offer a heightened risk for PPP[11–14] and others finding some specific risks.[15–17]

Parity

Numerous studies have found a higher risk for PPP in primiparous women.[13,15,17–19] Although some of that risk may exist because some women who experience PPP do not have further children (in one recent study, only 45% went on to have subsequent pregnancies),[16] that fact does not entirely explain the risk, for even those that restrict analysis to women who have had more than one pregnancy find a consistent risk for primiparous women.[15] Some of this risk may be due to the increased psychosocial stress of a first child, but some may also be due to unknown biological factors. Research has not yet illuminated whether time between pregnancies, pregnancies with different fathers, or sex of the fetus may affect a woman's risk; but these would be interesting areas to explore given the emerging literature on these areas for other pregnancy morbidities.[20–22]

Personal History of Bipolar Disorder

The strongest single risk factor for PPP is a personal history of bipolar disorder, with 20% to 30% of parous women with known bipolar disorder experiencing PPP.[23] Yet in a recent large study only 33% of women presenting with PPP had a prior psychiatric history, and of those only one-third had been diagnosed with bipolar disorder.[16] Although there is increasing evidence that some women with PPP will experience only puerperal episodes, most women who present with PPP as their first psychiatric episode will eventually meet the criteria for bipolar disorder, with one comprehensive study showing a risk of a subsequent nonpuerperal episode of 69%. A presentation of

PPP should, therefore, be considered bipolar disorder and treated as such until proved otherwise.

Family History/Genetic Factors

Although no specific genes that contribute to risk have been identified, there is strong evidence that puerperal psychotic episodes run in families.[24-26]

Preeclampsia

The clinical features and risk factors for PE overlap with those of PPP, including the strong risk of primiparity and the high risk of subsequent episodes. Evidence so far is inconclusive, however, with some studies finding no increased risk for PE in women with PPP.[27] One recent registry-based study did find a strong relationship between PE and first-onset postpartum psychiatric episodes, with an odds ratio approaching 5 in primiparous women, but did not distinguish between PPP and other types of post-partum psychiatric disturbance.[28] This subject remains an intriguing area for further research.

Sleep Disturbance

Sleep loss has long been recognized as a trigger for mania; in fact sleep deprivation can be used as an effective, if drastic, treatment of depression.[29-35] There has been very little research specifically on sleep deprivation and puerperal manic or psychotic episodes, though there has been an association noted between women who have longer labors or give birth in the middle of the night and the subsequent development of PPP.[36,37] A recent study found that women with known bipolar disorder who report that sleep disturbance is a common trigger for their manias are at heightened risk for episodes of PPP.[38] This finding was specific to PPP (as opposed to postpartum depression [PPD]) and indicates that future research in this area is warranted.

Immune Dysregulation

Perhaps the most intriguing recent evidence about the biological origins of PPP is the evidence for immune system dysregulation. Bergink and colleagues[39] have explored several areas of immune dysfunction in PPP[40] and found evidence for increased rates of autoimmune thyroiditis (present in 19% of subjects with PPP and only 5% of controls)[41] as well as failure of normal T-cell elevation, increased monocyte to nonmonocyte ratio, and significant upregulation of immune-related genes in subjects with PPP.[39,40] Kumar and colleagues[42] examined immune cell types by flow cytometry and found significant alterations in the number and type of T cells and natural killer cells in women with PPP. This subject is one of the most active areas of biological research on PPP.

Hormonal Change

Although the precipitous drop in estrogen and progesterone in the 24 hours following childbirth is a tempting candidate for the cause of postpartum psychiatric disorders, most studies have shown little difference in absolute levels of reproductive hormones between healthy women and those experiencing psychiatric symptoms.[43,44] Instead, certain women seem to have a vulnerability to hormonal fluctuation.[45] There has been very little research on hormonal contributors to PPP specifically. There have been case reports of women with PPP who have hypoparathyroidism[46] and Sheehan syndrome[47] and of the role of melatonin.[48] Some small trials and case reports have examined estrogen and progesterone for prevention or treatment of PPP, with mixed results for estrogen and no good evidence to support the use of progesterone (as summarized by Doucet and colleagues[49] in 2011). Although further research is clearly needed, at this time the evidence does not support the use of hormones either to treat or to prevent PPP.

SCREENING AND ASSESSMENT

There is no standardized set of questions or screening tool for PPP, and the diversity of presentation makes it difficult to create an algorithm for screening. The widely used Edinburgh Postnatal Depression Scale,[50] a 10-item self-report screen for PPD, will pick up symptoms of depression or anxiety; but it cannot distinguish between unipolar and bipolar depression nor can it assess symptoms of psychosis. There is also no completely standard set of laboratory tests because of the rarity of the disorder, but evidence about the biological cause has grown enough at this point to suggest a likely set of laboratory tests. **Boxes 5** and **6** outline the most important screening questions and laboratory tools.

DIFFERENTIAL DIAGNOSIS

PPP is one of 3 affective (mood) syndromes that can affect women in the postpartum. The baby blues affect 85% to 90% of women.[51–53] This syndrome is a self-limited syndrome of mood lability (up or down), tearfulness, and feeling overwhelmed, but without serious effects on the woman's functioning. It occurs within days of birth and is generally resolved within 2 weeks. It is unrelated to psychiatric history and requires no intervention other than support. PPD is a more serious disorder that can include low mood, anhedonia, and sometimes suicidality. It affects 10% to 20% of postpartum women.[54] The *Diagnostic and Statistical Manual of Mental Disorders* (*DSM*) defines it as a depressive episode "with peripartum onset,"[55] beginning in the third trimester or within 4 weeks post partum. Symptoms must last at least 2 weeks to qualify as a depressive episode; but any woman whose symptoms are severe and affect functioning and/or is suicidal, unable to function, or exhibits suicidality should be suspected of likely depression even if that time criterion has not been met. Although it often begins within the *DSM*-specified time period, many women will not present until later in the postpartum course. Women with PPD are often anxious[56]; postpartum women can also present with generalized anxiety disorder, a condition in which patients worry excessively about things across many domains of life.

Box 5
Important screening questions for patients and/or families

- Is this the patient's first psychiatric presentation?
- If she has a psychiatric history, is it of depression, mania, or both?
- Is there any family history of bipolar disorder?
- Has the patient been using any substances?
- Does the patient have thoughts of harming herself or the child? It is important to ask this in a nonjudgmental fashion: It can be very overwhelming to be a new mother. Sometimes women have scary thoughts; they might think about hurting themselves or hurting their babies. Has that ever happened to you?

Box 6
Important assessment tools

- Complete physical examination
- Neurologic examination
- Comprehensive metabolic panel
- Complete blood count
- Urinalysis
- Urine toxicology screen
- Thyroid stimulating hormone, free thyroxine (T4) and thyroid peroxidase antibodies
- Ammonia level
- If neurologic symptoms present, brain imaging and testing for limbic encephalitis

---

Perhaps the most difficult psychiatric condition to distinguish from PPP is postpartum obsessive-compulsive disorder (OCD). There is evidence of an increased risk of onset and flare of OCD during times of reproductive transition,[57,58] and it is important to distinguish between the frightening intrusive thoughts common in OCD (obsessions) and the delusions that characterize PPP. See **Table 1** for a description of these differences.

In addition to these psychiatric conditions, there are several medical conditions that must be considered in suspected cases of PPD. The waxing and waning of consciousness that is often seen is reminiscent of delirium, and delirium for medical causes (most commonly infection surrounding parturition) should be at the top of any clinician's differential. Tests of attention and cognitive function, such as the Mini-Mental State Examination and the Montreal Cognitive Assessment, can help to determine whether delirium is present, as can laboratory tests, including urinalysis and complete blood count. There have been several cases of autoimmune encephalitis presenting as PPD; postpartum abnormalities, such as Sheehan syndrome or flares of autoimmune diseases (such as lupus), can also have neuropsychiatric presentations.[59] See **Box 7** for a complete differential list.

Table 1
Obsessions versus delusions

Obsessions	Delusions
• Intrusive thoughts that are unwanted and horrifying to patients	• Fixed false belief
• Can be sexual, religious, or violent	• Content often bizarre or unusual; can also be sexual, religious, or violent
• Patient has no desire to act on these thoughts	• Patients may want to act on these thoughts or feel compelled to do so
• Thoughts cause considerable distress and patients may avoid things or engage in compulsive behavior (checking, seeking reassurance) to ease that distress	• Thoughts may not cause significant distress
• *Example: Mother has an intrusive thought about molesting her child while changing diapers; this horrifies her and she insists that her husband change all diapers.*	• *Example: Mother thinks her child has been cursed by the devil and that she must throw him or her out the window.*

> **Box 7**
> **Differential diagnosis for postpartum psychosis**
>
> - Baby blues
> - PPD
> - Generalized anxiety disorder
> - OCD
> - Delirium
> - Autoimmune encephalitis (ie, N-methyl-d-aspartate receptor)
> - Sheehan syndrome
> - Autoimmune flare (ie, neuropsychiatric symptoms of lupus)
> - Intoxication
> - Medication reaction (ie, steroid-induced mania)

MANAGEMENT
Treatment Setting

PPP is a psychiatric emergency that requires inpatient hospitalization. In much of the developed world, that hospitalization can take place in a dedicated mother-baby psychiatric unit, the type of facility that is deemed best practice in many countries.[60] These units, which were first established in the 1950s in the United Kingdom and in the 1970s and 1980s in Europe and Australia, promote mother-baby attachment during the period of treatment of severe mental illness in the postpartum period. Unfortunately, this is a concept that has yet to take hold in the United States, where there are no psychiatric units that permit babies to stay with their mothers. Many clinicians, whether obstetricians or psychiatrists, and many patients and families are, therefore, reluctant to seek hospitalization when it means a disruption of the mother-child bond and a disruption of breast-feeding. The severity of PPP, however, means that in the US treatment setting such separation is usually warranted. PPP is associated with high rates of both suicide and infanticide,[61] and treatment can occur most safely and rapidly in the context of inpatient hospitalization. Any obstetrician encountering a suspected case of PPP should, therefore, seek immediate psychiatric consultation (if inpatient) or refer patients to the emergency department (if outpatient).

Pharmacologic Treatment

The rarity of PPP, and the ethical difficulty of randomizing postpartum patients experiencing a psychiatric emergency, means that the evidence about treatments relies on data from small observational studies only. A 2011 review identified 10 studies of pharmacologic interventions to prevent PPP and 17 to treat it.[49] Approaches studied included antipsychotics, mood stabilizers, hormones, propranolol, and electroconvulsive therapy (ECT), all in either case reports or small observational studies. Some evidence of efficacy was found for all approaches except hormone therapy. The strongest evidence was found for ECT, for which 3 small studies reported improvement for all women undergoing ECT for PPD.

Since that time, the group of Bergink and colleagues,[62] in the Netherlands, has published numerous larger studies on both the cause and treatment of PPP. In the largest treatment trial to date, this group followed 64 women from admission for PPP through

9 months post partum, following a 3-step treatment algorithm. Step 1 was lorazepam at bedtime for 3 days; 4 out of 64 subjects remitted at this stage. Step 2 was the addition of an antipsychotic (usually haloperidol 2–6 mg daily) on day 4; 12 of the remaining 60 subjects remitted at this stage. Step 3 was the addition of lithium after 2 weeks of nonresponse to steps 1 and 2, to a targeted lithium serum level between 0.8 and 1.2 mmol/L; 47 of the remaining 48 subjects remitted at this stage (with the remaining patient discharged against medical advice before remission). Step 4 was ECT after 12 weeks of nonresponse to steps 1, 2, and 3; no subjects advanced to this stage. The investigators tapered off benzodiazepines and antipsychotics after symptom remission and continued lithium (or antipsychotics if patients responded without lithium) for 9 months, with nearly 80% of patients retaining full remission at 9 months post partum.

This timetable for treatment is unrealistic in US treatment settings, where the average acute psychiatric hospitalization lasts only 10 days.[63] Because 98% of subjects in Bergink and colleague's[62] study responded to lithium, most perinatal psychiatrists recommend the early addition of lithium. Because there is a high rate of recurrence (more than 54% recurrence of PPP in one recent study),[16] prophylaxis with lithium is recommended for subsequent postpartum episodes. This recommendation is based on the treatment algorithm of Bergink and colleagues,[62] as described earlier; in that study, only 10% of those maintained on lithium throughout the follow-up period relapsed. Another study of women maintained on lithium throughout pregnancy found a relapse rate of 11% during pregnancy and 29% in the postpartum period for any mood episode, including PPP.[64] (There has not yet been a study, however, that has examined the efficacy of prophylaxis specifically for subsequent pregnancies in women who have experienced PPP.) Although there are risks to using lithium in both pregnancy and breastfeeding,[65,66] those risks are much lower than was once thought and for many women will be outweighed by the risks of PPP (which include suicide, infanticide, poor mother-child bonding, and subsequent PPD with consequences for child development). See **Box 8** for a recommended treatment algorithm.

Psychosocial Supports

Given the severity of symptoms, pharmacologic treatment is always necessary in PPP. Low socioeconomic status and acute stressors increase women's risk for PPD[11] but do not affect the risk for PPP, and evidence concerning psychosocial treatments is weak. Yet family and other psychosocial support is crucial for recovery in PPP. Regardless of the type of mood symptoms involved (manic, depressive, or both),

---

Box 8
Treatment recommendations for acute postpartum psychosis

- Benzodiazepine (lorazepam 0.5–1.5 mg 3 times a day)
- Antipsychotic (high potency preferred, haloperidol 2–6 mg or olanzapine 10–15 mg)
- Lithium (to achieve serum level of 0.8–1.2 mmol/L)
- Tapered benzodiazepine and antipsychotic once symptom remission achieved
- Continued lithium monotherapy for 9 months (can lower to achieve serum level of 0.6–0.8 after symptom remission if severe side effects)
- For future pregnancies: prophylactic lithium monotherapy beginning during pregnancy or immediately post partum

insomnia is a prominent feature of the illness; sleep hygiene interventions are crucial. Support for the other parent, if any, is also important, as is specific feedback designed to improve the mother-baby interaction. Some groups have used video feedback, individual interventions by nursing staff, or baby massage.[62,67]

Patient and Child Safety

Perhaps the scariest aspect of PPP for the practicing obstetrician is how to determine whether patients are a danger to themselves or their children. Because rates of suicide and infanticide are high,[61] it is important to assess this and to remember that it is always better to err on the side of extra caution. Women with psychiatric illness can and do make excellent mothers, but those with acute PPP may be in danger of harming their children either deliberately or through neglect in the throes of illness. Involve psychiatry if at all possible in making this determination; it is easy for nonspecialists to misinterpret intrusive, obsessional thoughts for psychotic thoughts.

SUMMARY

PPP is a devastating complication of childbirth that carries high risks for both mother and child. Any suspected case requires a thorough psychiatric evaluation as soon as possible. The rarity of the disorder makes it difficult to study; the amount we do not know about risk factors, prevention, and treatment is large. Nevertheless, there are certain key clinical features and risk factors of which the practicing obstetrician can and should be aware:

- Remember that women with known bipolar disorder are at greatest risk but that only one-third of women who present with PPP will have a prior psychiatric history.
- Remember to ask all patients about their personal and family history of bipolar disorder.
- Remember that primiparous women are at the highest risk.
- Always ask about sleep disturbance: Although all new mothers will have disrupted sleep, those who are not able to sleep when they have the opportunity should raise a red flag.
- Always ask, in a neutral and nonjudgmental way, about the woman's thoughts of harming herself or the child; remember that the important distinction is whether a woman is disturbed or horrified by these thoughts (indicating that they may be obsessions).
- Remember that PPP is a psychiatric emergency; if you suspect it, patients must have a psychiatric evaluation as soon as possible (in the emergency department if necessary).

REFERENCES

1. Jones I, Chandra PS, Dazzan P, et al. Bipolar disorder, affective psychosis, and schizophrenia in pregnancy and the post-partum period. Lancet 2014;384(9956): 1789–99.
2. Sit D, Rothschild AJ, Wisner KL. A review of postpartum psychosis. J Womens Health (Larchmt) 2006;15(4):352–68.
3. Hatters Friedman S, Sorrentino R. Commentary: postpartum psychosis, infanticide, and insanity–implications for forensic psychiatry. J Am Acad Psychiatry Law 2012;40(3):326–32.

4. Spinelli MG. Infanticide: psychosocial and legal perspectives on mothers who kill. Washington, DC: American Psychiatric Publishing; 2008.

5. Marcé L-V. Traité de la folie des femmes enceintes, des nouvelles accouchées, et des nourrices. Paris (France): J.B. Ballière; 1858.

6. Kendell RE, Chalmers JC, Platz C. Epidemiology of puerperal psychoses. Br J Psychiatry 1987;150:662–73.

7. Valdimarsdóttir U, Hultman CM, Harlow B, et al. Psychotic illness in first-time mothers with no previous psychiatric hospitalizations: a population-based study. PLoS Med 2009;6(2):e13.

8. Klompenhouwer J, van Hulst A, Tulen J, et al. The clinical features of postpartum psychoses. Eur Psychiatry 1995;10(7):355–67.

9. Kamperman AM, Veldman-Hoek MJ, Wesseloo R, et al. Phenotypical characteristics of postpartum psychosis: a clinical cohort study. Bipolar Disord 2017; 19(6):450–7.

10. Esquirol, Etienne. Des maladies mentales: considérées sous les rapports médical, hygiénique et médico-legal. Paris: J. B. Balliere; 1838.

11. Meltzer-Brody S, Maegbaek ML, Medland SE, et al. Obstetrical, pregnancy and socio-economic predictors for new-onset severe postpartum psychiatric disorders in primiparous women. Psychol Med 2017;47(8):1427–41.

12. Kumar R, Marks M, Platz C, et al. Clinical survey of a psychiatric mother and baby unit: characteristics of 100 consecutive admissions. J Affect Disord 1995;33(1): 11–22.

13. Videbech PB, Gouliaev GH. Prognosis of the onset of postpartum psychosis. Demographic, obstetric and psychiatric factors. Ugeskr Laeger 1996;158(21): 2970–4 [in Danish].

14. Munk-Olsen T, Laursen TM, Pedersen CB, et al. New parents and mental disorders: a population-based register study. JAMA 2006;296(21): 2582–9.

15. Blackmore ER, Jones I, Doshi M, et al. Obstetric variables associated with bipolar affective puerperal psychosis. Br J Psychiatry 2006;188:32–6.

16. Blackmore ER, Rubinow DR, O'Connor TG, et al. Reproductive outcomes and risk of subsequent illness in women diagnosed with postpartum psychosis. Bipolar Disord 2013;15(4):394–404.

17. Paffenbarger R. Motherhood and mental illness. London: Academic Press; 1982.

18. Munk-Olsen T, Jones I, Laursen TM. Birth order and postpartum psychiatric disorders. Bipolar Disord 2014;16(3):300–7.

19. Di Florio A, Jones L, Forty L, et al. Mood disorders and parity - a clue to the aetiology of the postpartum trigger. J Affect Disord 2014;152–154:334–9.

20. Andersen LB, Jørgensen JS, Herse F, et al. The association between angiogenic markers and fetal sex: implications for preeclampsia research. J Reprod Immunol 2016;117:24–9.

21. Zheng Q, Deng Y, Zhong S, et al. Human chorionic gonadotropin, fetal sex and risk of hypertensive disorders of pregnancy: a nested case-control study. Pregnancy Hypertens 2016;6(1):17–21.

22. Katsi V, Felekos I, Siristatidis C, et al. Preeclampsia: what does the father have to do with it? Curr Hypertens Rep 2015;17(8):60.

23. Di Florio A, Forty L, Gordon-Smith K, et al. Perinatal episodes across the mood disorder spectrum. JAMA Psychiatry 2013;70(2):168–75.

24. Jones I, Craddock N. Familiality of the puerperal trigger in bipolar disorder: results of a family study. Am J Psychiatry 2001;158(6):913–7.

25. Jones I, Craddock N. Do puerperal psychotic episodes identify a more familial subtype of bipolar disorder? Results of a family history study. Psychiatr Genet 2002;12(3):177–80.
26. Jones I, Hamshere M, Nangle JM, et al. Bipolar affective puerperal psychosis: genome-wide significant evidence for linkage to chromosome 16. Am J Psychiatry 2007;164(7):1099–104.
27. Bergink V, Lambregtse-van den Berg MP, Koorengevel KM, et al. First-onset psychosis occurring in the postpartum period: a prospective cohort study. J Clin Psychiatry 2011;72(11):1531–7.
28. Bergink V, Laursen TM, Johannsen BM, et al. Pre-eclampsia and first-onset postpartum psychiatric episodes: a Danish population-based cohort study. Psychol Med 2015;45(16):3481–9.
29. Benedetti F. Antidepressant chronotherapeutics for bipolar depression. Dialogues Clin Neurosci 2012;14(4):401–11.
30. Wirz-Justice A, Benedetti F, Berger M, et al. Chronotherapeutics (light and wake therapy) in affective disorders. Psychol Med 2005;35(7):939–44.
31. Wehr TA. Sleep loss: a preventable cause of mania and other excited states. J Clin Psychiatry 1989;50(Suppl):8–16 [discussion 45–7].
32. Wehr TA. Sleep-loss as a possible mediator of diverse causes of mania. Br J Psychiatry 1991;159:576–8.
33. Wehr TA, Goodwin FK, Wirz-Justice A, et al. 48-hour sleep-wake cycles in manic-depressive illness: naturalistic observations and sleep deprivation experiments. Arch Gen Psychiatry 1982;39(5):559–65.
34. Wehr TA, Sack DA, Rosenthal NE. Sleep reduction as a final common pathway in the genesis of mania. Am J Psychiatry 1987;144(2):201–4.
35. Bauer M, Grof P, Rasgon N, et al. Temporal relation between sleep and mood in patients with bipolar disorder. Bipolar Disord 2006;8(2):160–7.
36. Sharma V, Smith A, Khan M. The relationship between duration of labour, time of delivery, and puerperal psychosis. J Affect Disord 2004;83(2–3):215–20.
37. Lewis KJ, Foster RG, Jones IR. Is sleep disruption a trigger for postpartum psychosis? Br J Psychiatry 2016;208(5):409–11.
38. Lewis KJS, Di Florio A, Forty L, et al. Mania triggered by sleep loss and risk of postpartum psychosis in women with bipolar disorder. J Affect Disord 2018;225:624–9.
39. Bergink V, Burgerhout KM, Weigelt K, et al. Immune system dysregulation in first-onset postpartum psychosis. Biol Psychiatry 2013;73(10):1000–7.
40. Weigelt K, Bergink V, Burgerhout KM, et al. Down-regulation of inflammation-protective microRNAs 146a and 212 in monocytes of patients with postpartum psychosis. Brain Behav Immun 2013;29:147–55.
41. Bergink V, Kushner SA, Pop V, et al. Prevalence of autoimmune thyroid dysfunction in postpartum psychosis. Br J Psychiatry 2011;198(4):264–8.
42. Kumar MM, Venkataswamy MM, Sathyanarayanan G, et al. Immune system aberrations in postpartum psychosis: an immunophenotyping study from a tertiary care neuropsychiatric hospital in India. J Neuroimmunol 2017;310:8–13.
43. Schiller CE, Meltzer-Brody S, Rubinow DR. The role of reproductive hormones in postpartum depression. CNS Spectr 2015;20(1):48–59.
44. Yim IS, Tanner Stapleton LR, Guardino CM, et al. Biological and psychosocial predictors of postpartum depression: systematic review and call for integration. Annu Rev Clin Psychol 2015;11:99–137.

45. Bloch M, Schmidt PJ, Danaceau M, et al. Effects of gonadal steroids in women with a history of postpartum depression. Am J Psychiatry 2000;157(6): 924–30.
46. Patil NJ, Yadav SS, Gokhale YA, et al. Primary hypoparathyroidism: psychosis in postpartum period. J Assoc Physicians India 2010;58:506–8.
47. Kale K, Nihalani N, Karnik N, et al. Postpartum psychosis in a case of Sheehan's syndrome. Indian J Psychiatry 1999;41(1):70–2.
48. Anderson G. The role of melatonin in post-partum psychosis and depression associated with bipolar disorder. J Perinat Med 2010;38(6):585–7.
49. Doucet S, Jones I, Letourneau N, et al. Interventions for the prevention and treatment of postpartum psychosis: a systematic review. Arch Womens Ment Health 2011;14(2):89–98.
50. Cox JL, Holden JM, Sagovsky R. Detection of postnatal depression. development of the 10-item Edinburgh postnatal depression scale. Br J Psychiatry 1987;150: 782–6.
51. Payne JL, Palmer JT, Joffe H. A reproductive subtype of depression: conceptualizing models and moving toward etiology. Harv Rev Psychiatry 2009;17(2): 72–86.
52. Campbell SB, Cohn JF. Prevalence and correlates of postpartum depression in first-time mothers. J Abnorm Psychol 1991;100(4):594–9.
53. Frank E, Kupfer DJ, Jacob M, et al. Pregnancy-related affective episodes among women with recurrent depression. Am J Psychiatry 1987;144(3):288–93.
54. Yonkers KA, Vigod S, Ross LE. Diagnosis, pathophysiology, and management of mood disorders in pregnant and postpartum women. Obstet Gynecol 2011; 117(4):961–77.
55. American Psychiatric Association. Diagnostic and statistical manual of mental disorders. 5th edition. Arlington (VA): American Psychiatric Publishing; 2013.
56. Schofield CA, Battle CL, Howard M, et al. Symptoms of the anxiety disorders in a perinatal psychiatric sample: a chart review. J Nerv Ment Dis 2014;202(2): 154–60.
57. Forray A, Focseneanu M, Pittman B, et al. Onset and exacerbation of obsessive-compulsive disorder in pregnancy and the postpartum period. J Clin Psychiatry 2010;71(8):1061–8.
58. Labad J, Menchón JM, Alonso P, et al. Female reproductive cycle and obsessive-compulsive disorder. J Clin Psychiatry 2005;66(4):428–35 [quiz: 546].
59. Jafri K, Patterson SL, Lanata C. Central nervous system manifestations of systemic lupus erythematosus. Rheum Dis Clin North Am 2017;43(4): 531–45.
60. Connellan K, Bartholomaeus C, Due C, et al. A systematic review of research on psychiatric mother-baby units. Arch Womens Ment Health 2017;20(3):373–88.
61. Spinelli MG. Postpartum psychosis: detection of risk and management. Am J Psychiatry 2009;166(4):405–8.
62. Bergink V, Burgerhout KM, Koorengevel KM, et al. Treatment of psychosis and mania in the postpartum period. Am J Psychiatry 2015;172(2):115–23.
63. Lee S, Rothbard AB, Noll EL. Length of inpatient stay of persons with serious mental illness: effects of hospital and regional characteristics. Psychiatr Serv 2012;63(9):889–95.
64. Rosso G, Albert U, Di Salvo G, et al. Lithium prophylaxis during pregnancy and the postpartum period in women with lithium-responsive bipolar I disorder. Arch Womens Ment Health 2016;19(2):429–32.

65. Patorno E, Huybrechts KF, Bateman BT, et al. Lithium use in pregnancy and the risk of cardiac malformations. N Engl J Med 2017;376(23):2245-54.
66. Haskey C, Galbally M. Mood stabilizers in pregnancy and child developmental outcomes: a systematic review. Aust N Z J Psychiatry 2017;51(11): 1087-97.
67. Meltzer-Brody S, Brandon AR, Pearson B, et al. Evaluating the clinical effectiveness of a specialized perinatal psychiatry inpatient unit. Arch Womens Ment Health 2014;17(2):107-13.

Identification and Treatment of Peripartum Anxiety Disorders

Katherine E. Williams, MD[a], Hristina Koleva, MD[b],*

KEYWORDS

• Anxiety • Anxiety disorders • Perinatal • Peripartum • Screening • Treatment

KEY POINTS

- Anxiety disorders in pregnancy and the postpartum period are common and can present independently or together with depression.
- Specific anxiety disorders have characteristic presentations and clinicians will benefit from familiarizing with their criteria. Specific disorders require tailored treatment.
- Women should be screened for anxiety symptoms during pregnancy and at postpartum follow-up, but guidelines are limited. General screening tools for anxiety can be used.
- Prompt treatment with first-line evidence–based therapies, including selective serotonin reuptake inhibitors/serotonin norepinephrine reuptake inhibitors and cognitive behavioral therapy, is indicated in collaboration with a mental health specialist.
- Benzodiazepines may be used at low doses and short-term. Decisions about risk and benefits of medications should be discussed on an individual basis.

INTRODUCTION

Anxiety disorders are the most common psychiatric disorders that affect women during the childbearing age.[1] The peripartum period is a particularly stressful time that increases the risk for some women to develop new-onset or have an exacerbation of preexisting anxiety symptoms and disorders. Frequently, anxiety accompanies symptoms of depression, and many times anxiety symptoms are the primary reason for mental health referral in expectant or new mothers. Anxiety symptoms during pregnancy are one of the strongest risk factors for postpartum depression.[2] Moreover, in many cases anxiety complaints are the sole presentation, and they are particularly

Disclosure Statement: Dr K.E. Williams and Dr H. Koleva do not have any commercial or financial conflicts of interest and any funding sources related to this article.
[a] Department of Psychiatry and Behavioral Sciences, Stanford University School of Medicine, 401 Quarry Road, Stanford, CA 94305-5717, USA; [b] Department of Psychiatry, University of Iowa, 200 Hawkins Drive, Iowa City, IA 52242, USA
* Corresponding author.
E-mail address: hristina-koleva@uiowa.edu

Obstet Gynecol Clin N Am 45 (2018) 469–481
https://doi.org/10.1016/j.ogc.2018.04.001
0889-8545/18/© 2018 Elsevier Inc. All rights reserved.

obgyn.theclinics.com

debilitating not only for the patient but also for the mother–infant relationship and the family unit as a whole.

Although perinatal depression has received growing attention, research, screening, and treatment of anxiety in the perinatal period have lagged behind. In a positive direction, the literature on the subject has certainly expanded over the last decade; still there is a need for comprehensive review.[3]

This article first presents information about the prevalence, adverse effects, differential diagnosis, and risk factors for perinatal anxiety disorders. The authors also recommend a method for identification, and finally, reviews current treatments for anxiety disorders in the perinatal period.

PREVALENCE AND ADVERSE EFFECTS

It is normal for expectant or new mothers to report anxiety symptoms. Up to two-thirds of women experience worries, most commonly consisting of fear about having an abnormal baby; complications during pregnancy or during birth; their ability to care for the baby, including breastfeeding and soothing the infant when crying; as well as concerns about body changes, partner relationships, job performance, finances, cleanliness etc.[4] It is only when the worries and anxiety symptoms interfere with daily functioning and cause significant distress that they are considered abnormal and may be part of an anxiety disorder. It is hypothesized that anxiety symptoms are correlated with the many biological changes that occur in women's bodies during pregnancy, including elevations of heart rate, changes in hormone levels, shallow breathing due to abdominal enlargement,[5] which can all lead to heightened sensitivity to normal and abnormal life stressors. Women with personal or family history of anxiety disorders are particularly vulnerable to these changes.

Studies on the incidence and prevalence of anxiety disorders during pregnancy and the postpartum period have used various methodologies and patient settings.[6–16] A summary of data derived from some of the most notable studies is presented in **Table 1**. Despite the inconsistencies in studies' methodologies and patient populations, it is clear that anxiety disorders in the perinatal period are common and occur with equal frequency in the antepartum and the postpartum period.

A major concern for pregnant women who present with anxiety disorders in the medical setting is the impact that these disorders can have on the wellbeing of the mother and the baby. Multiple studies have reported increased rate of peripartum complications in women who have anxiety symptoms and anxiety disorders, including preeclampsia, hypertension during pregnancy, low birth weight, premature delivery,

Table 1 Prevalence estimates of peripartum anxiety disorders		
Disorder	**Antepartum**	**Postpartum**
Generalized Anxiety Disorder	10%[4,7]	7%–8%[9]
Obsessive Compulsive Disorder	1.2%–5.2%[6–8]	0.7%–4% at 6–8 wk 4% at 6 mo < 1% at 12 mo[10]
Panic Disorder	1.4%–9.8%[11]	0.5%–2.9% at 6–10 wk[9,12]
Social Anxiety	2%–6.4%[4,13]	4.1% at 8 wk 2.3% at 6 mo 1.7% at 12 mo[9]
Posttraumatic Stress Disorder, Childbirth-related	Unknown	0.8%–4.6% (self-report)[14,15]

prolonged labor, postpartum hemorrhage, and other adverse outcomes.[17] In addition, anxious women are more likely than nonanxious women to report negative hospital experiences, lower perceived ability to take care of the baby, and have doubts about their parenting skills.[18] They are also at increased risk for postpartum depression.[19] Negative infant and child outcomes have also been reported, including low-birth weight, impaired mother–infant relationship, blunted cognitive and motor development, increased risk for attention-deficit/hyperactivity disorder, and other emotional and behavioral problems in children from birth up to 4 to 8 years of age.[20,21] In summary, all of the studies suggest a potential benefit of screening women for anxiety in the period both before and after giving birth, with the goal of appropriate identification and adequate treatment to reduce the risks associated with anxiety disorders.

DIFFERENTIAL DIAGNOSIS

Anxiety disorders are fully described in the psychiatric Diagnostic and Statistical Manual (DSM). According to its latest version, DSM-V, the most common anxiety disorders are generalized anxiety disorder (GAD), obsessive compulsive disorder (OCD), panic disorder, and social anxiety disorder. Posttraumatic stress disorder (PTSD) is a rare but very distressing condition that can also present with anxiety symptoms.

Generalized Anxiety Disorder

Frequent worrying is a normal experience in pregnant and postpartum women. About two-thirds of women report worries about "abnormal baby," and about half of pregnant women are concerned about potential pregnancy-related complications. Other common worries are about appearance, particularly weight gain, finances, cleanliness, breastfeeding etc. When worries occupy more than 50% of daily life and interfere with functioning and/or cause significant distress, a diagnosis of generalized anxiety disorder is considered. It is also high on the diagnostic radar if the patient cannot be reassured about her concerns, when the worries cannot be controlled, or when there is a lack of identifiable trigger for the anxiety symptoms. In about half of the cases, there is comorbidity with major depression or subsyndromal depression.[9] In contrast to depression, women who experience anxiety describe feeling as "jittery," on edge, hyperactive, and exhausted by the end of the day. They also frequently check on the baby and present to the pediatrician or primary physician promptly or frequently.

Panic Disorder

Panic attacks are common experiences in the general population. Panic attacks usually have an abrupt onset and reach a peak within minutes and typically include feelings of intense fear, palpitations, shortness of breath, sweating, shaking, numbness and tingling, etc. Panic attacks that are frequent, occur regularly for more than 1 month, and lead to severe distress and changes in behavior indicate panic disorder (DSM-V). Panic attacks in pregnant and postpartum women are similar in presentation to panic attacks that occur in nonpregnant women. Panic disorder can lead to agoraphobia, which is the avoidance of public places, and can lead to social isolation and dependence on others. Panic disorder in mothers is frequently associated with guilt and shame and can significantly impair woman's self-esteem and confidence in taking care of the baby. Moreover, women with panic disorder have increased help-seeking behavior, including frequent perinatal medical checks and emergency room visits. The impairment in the mother's functioning can also pose significant strain on the schedules and functioning of other family members, especially the partner.

Obsessive Compulsive Disorder

OCD is a rare disorder in the general population that is characterized by obsessions—recurrent, unwanted, inappropriate and intrusive thoughts, images or urges, and compulsions—repetitive behaviors (washing, checking) or mental acts (counting, repeating words), performed in response to an obsession. Intrusive thoughts are common in the pregnancy and postpartum period, as high as 91% of new mothers report them.[10] The theme usually revolves around concerns about possible harm to the baby, such as dropping or suffocating the baby, and fear of contamination. Sexual thoughts and fear of hurting the baby can also occur, and are disturbing for women, accompanied by shame and guilt. When OCD symptoms are severe they can lead to avoidance of the newborn and increased help-seeking behavior, such as the mother delegating care for the baby to their partner or other family members. Compulsions in mothers with OCD are rare. The obsessions can co-occur with symptoms of depression in about 50% of the cases.[9] OCD should be differentiated from postpartum psychosis, in which mothers have thoughts about harming the baby, which the mother does not view as inappropriate or distressful. Postpartum psychosis is considered a psychiatric emergency, whereas postpartum OCD can be successfully managed in the outpatient setting with therapy and medications.

Social Anxiety Disorder

Social anxiety disorder has been generally overlooked in the literature, despite occurring almost as commonly as GAD (see **Table 1**). Women who present with perinatal social anxiety usually have it before the pregnancy. They experience symptoms of avoidance of social situations, anxiety about public performance, and fear of new experiences. Sometimes, clinically significant social anxiety has new onset after childbirth[9] and can challenge the adaptation of new mothers in the community. Specifically, it can lead to strained relationship with the partner, difficulty adjusting to work following maternity leave, and lower life satisfaction.

Posttraumatic Stress Disorder

Although up to 75% of women report fear associated with labor and delivery, PTSD related to child-birth is rare. Women who have traumatic experience during labor and delivery can develop PTSD when they fear that they or their newborn may die or are at risk for serious harm. The typical symptoms include the following:

1. Reexperiencing of the trauma (flashbacks and nightmares)
2. Avoidance, presenting as inadequate baby care, missing obstetrician-gynecologist (OBGYN) appointments
3. Numbing: presenting as estrangement from others, insecure attachment with the baby
4. Increased arousal: being easily startled by baby cues, for example, baby crying

Personal history of traumatic events and abuse increases the risk for complicated delivery[22] and PTSD. There is high comorbidity of PTSD and postpartum major depression, up to 65% according to some reports.[23]

RISK FACTORS FOR PERINATAL ANXIETY DISORDERS

Medically high-risk pregnancies increase the risk for the development of perinatal anxiety disorders (**Table 2**).[17] Women who have given birth to preterm infants have also been identified as being at high risk for the development of anxiety disorders, especially PTSD.[31]

Table 2
Risk factors for perinatal anxiety disorders

Anxiety Disorder	Perinatal Risk Factors
Panic Disorder	Prepregnancy panic disorder[24] Psychosocial stress[25] Recent interpersonal violence[26]
Generalized Anxiety Disorder (GAD)	Prepregnancy GAD[27]
Obsessive Compulsive Disorder	Family history OCD[8] Avoidant and obsessive compulsive personality disorders[8] Premenstrual dysphoric disorder[28] Postpartum depression[29]
Social Phobia	Unknown
Posttraumatic Stress Disorder	Traumatic childbirth experiences[14,24] Recent interpersonal violence[14,24] Childhood adverse experiences[30]

SUMMARY: RISK FACTORS FOR ANXIETY DISORDERS—WHAT TO LOOK FOR IN THE CLINICAL HISTORY

Recognition of patients at risk for perinatal anxiety disorders may be difficult. Many women do not want to reveal their past diagnosis of an anxiety disorder, and their worries may be interpreted as normal anxiety by both the woman and her practitioner. Questions to ask in the clinical interview include the following:

- Have you ever been diagnosed or treated for an anxiety disorder? If so, what sort of treatment: medication (what kind and dose) and/or psychotherapy (type and frequency)?
- How stressed are you feeling right now? Are you having significant problems with your family/partner/housing/finances?
- Is anyone hurting you at home right now?
- Did your past pregnancies and deliveries turn out as you expected? Did you suffer any complications or traumas?

SCREENING FOR PERINATAL ANXIETY DISORDERS

Multiple national health organizations have recommended screening all pregnant and postpartum women for mood disorders. However, despite the growing recognition of the high prevalence of perinatal anxiety disorders, no comparable screening recommendations have been made for these disorders. Currently, there is no consensus regarding specific anxiety measures, frequency of sampling, or at-risk perinatal groups in whom clinicians should focus screening efforts on.

EPDS AS A PERINATAL SCREENING TOOL

Other useful screening tools for perinatal anxiety disorders are listed in **Table 3**. The EPDS-3A (3 questions from the 10-item measure) is now recognized as an effective screening tool for anxiety.[32] By focusing on questions 3 ("I have blamed myself unnecessarily when things went wrong"), 4 ("I have been anxious or worried for no good reason"), and 5 (I have felt scared or panicky for no good reason"), the clinician can screen for a comorbid or primary perinatal anxiety disorder. Scores on the EPDS 3-A greater than or equal to 5 have been suggested as cut-off score for further evaluation

Table 3
Useful screening tools and questions for perinatal anxiety disorders

Anxiety Disorder	Measure	Recommendations
Generalized Anxiety Disorder (GAD)	GAD-7[33]	GAD-7>10 evaluate for GAD with clinical interview All patients with history of GAD should complete GAD-7 during pregnancy and postpartum
Panic Disorder (PD)	Severity measure PD-adult[34]	Administer severity measure PD if preexisting PD diagnosis Mental health referral if medically unexplained acute episodes of shortness of breath, tachycardia, dizziness, paresthesias, feelings of dread, panic
Obsessive Compulsive Disorder	Perinatal obsessive compulsive scale (POCS)[35]	Administer POCS to women with history of OCD Ask all women is they have unwanted/intrusive thoughts or compulsive behaviors: "It is not uncommon for new mothers to experience intrusive, unwanted thoughts that they might harm their baby. Have any such thoughts occurred to you?"[36]
Posttraumatic Stress Disorder	Perinatal Posttraumatic Stress Disorder Questionnaire (PPQ)[37,38] Childbirth-specific version of the Posttraumatic Stress Symptom Scale-Self Report Version (PSS-SR)[39]	Administer PPQ or PSS-SR to women with a history of traumatic birth experiences, childhood trauma, interpersonal violence

and treatment of anxiety.[32] All pregnant patients and postpartum patients should be screened at first evaluation, and before delivery with the EPDS, and the EPDS 3-A score should be calculated. Patients with medically complicated pregnancies or preterm infants should be screened more frequently as they are at high risk (**Table 3**).

For OBGYNs with a close collaboration with a mental health professional, referral for patients identified at risk and currently symptomatic perinatal anxiety patients is indicated. Embedded care—the colocation of perinatal mental health specialists in obstetrics and gynecology clinics—facilitates this collaborative care model.[40]

TREATMENT CONSIDERATIONS
Psychotherapy

Panic disorder and generalized anxiety disorder
Treatment studies of perinatal anxiety disorders are limited.[24,41] Cognitive behavior therapy (CBT) is often described as a treatment of choice for panic disorder, generalized anxiety disorder, and obsessive compulsive disorder in pregnancy; however, to date, no large perinatal CBT anxiety treatment trials exist. There is only one case report for panic disorder[42] and a prevention trial for generalized anxiety disorder.[43]

Several trials of mindfulness-based interventions for generalized anxiety symptoms in pregnancy are being developed, and early reports are promising.

Obsessive compulsive disorder

CBT is a well-established evidence-based treatment of OCD in the general population[44] and positive case reports exist in the perinatal literature,[45,46] as well as a small intensive CBT trial for OCD.[47] Therefore, CBT should also be first-line treatment of mild-moderate OCD in the perinatal population and should be used in combination with medications such as selective serotonin reuptake inhibitors (SSRIs) for patients with severe symptoms. It is important to create a trusting relationship with the patient in order to uncover the obsessions, because many women may consider their obsessions to be too unacceptable to reveal them. Through eliciting the specific thoughts, response prevention and exposure components of CBT can be developed with an experienced therapist. It is very important for the clinician to provide a supportive atmosphere for the woman with OCD and to encourage her to bring her partner/family in for education. Several helpful OCD workbooks are available, including perinatal-specific, which explain how to support the patient with OCD.[48]

Posttraumatic stress disorder

Debriefing interventions, which include a health care professional (nurse, physician, psychologist, or social worker) reviewing the traumatic event with the patient very soon after the event has occurred, have not been shown to prevent perinatal PTSD[49] so it is not currently recommended as a primary treatment and prevention intervention. Nevertheless, obstetric personnel are encouraged to provide support and empathy to women who have had complicated deliveries and to allow them to ask questions about the event, because negative subjective birth experience is a predictor for PTSD,[50] and support from hospital staff has been shown to be helpful and may be protective factors to decrease the risk of PTSD.[51]

Trauma-focused psychotherapy by an experienced therapist is recommended for treatment of PTSD in the general population[52]; yet, despite the prevalence of perinatal PTSD, there have been no randomized controlled trials. Nevertheless, trauma-focused therapy by an experienced therapist is indicated for patients suffering from perinatal PTSD. Cognitive processing therapy and prolonged exposure include cognitive restructuring and hierarchical exposure therapy. Relaxation training and mindfulness meditation helps with the autonomic hyperarousal, and narrative therapy can engage the patient in reworking the memories, making greater sense of the trauma and creating a new, more self-compassionate narrative.

Social phobia

No studies have been completed for treatment of social phobia in pregnancy and postpartum.[24] Given that social phobia may interfere with mothers communicating and interfacing effectively with health care professionals and future school/day care providers, this is an area of treatment study in need of attention. In the general population, social phobia treatment with CBT is very effective and is the treatment of choice.[53]

MEDICATIONS
Antidepressants During Pregnancy

Panic disorder and generalized anxiety disorder psychopharmacology

If women are suffering from multiple panic attacks a day, the potential risk of medication may be less than the potential risk of ongoing autonomic nervous system hyperarousal. Severe GAD symptoms, especially those associated with autonomic nervous system instability may also be associated with pregnancy complications. There is extensive evidence basis for the treatment of both GAD and panic disorder with SSRIs, serotonin norepinephrine reuptake inhibitors (SNRIs), and tricyclic antidepressants (TCAs) in the general population; their use in perinatal population is extrapolated from this literature and to date, the perinatal anxiety studies are of small sample size and not placebo controlled. No comparison studies of antidepressants in perinatal anxiety disorders have been completed, and choice of antidepressant should be based on previous history of antidepressant efficacy, safety profile,[54] and side effect profile.

Because many pregnant patients prefer psychotherapy to medication[55] and pregnant anxious patients are especially preoccupied with safety concerns, the decision to initiate medications for panic or generalized anxiety disorder is often a difficult one. It is recommended that patients clarify their most distressing symptoms and that physician and patient partner track these symptoms through measures previously described. It is also recommended that the patient bring in her partner, if appropriate, as many women are conflicted about medication because their partner or important people in their lives oppose them. Psychoeducation about medications and the risks of untreated anxiety for the partner or family members can enhance family acceptable of this treatment approach and decrease the stress and guilt the patient feels about initiating medication.

For panic and generalized anxiety disorder patients in the general population, especially those with panic disorder, it is useful to start SSRIs at a lower dose than might be started in major depression, because of risk of exacerbating anxiety symptoms. SSRIs are preferred over SNRIs in the perinatal population because of more extensive safety studies, unless the patient has a previous history of nonresponse to SSRIs, and the SNRI has been the only medication in the past to help the patient. If an SNRI is used, it is important to follow blood pressure carefully.

TCAs were used in the largest clinical trial of treatment of panic disorder in pregnant women; 75% of women responded to imipramine at low doses (10–40 mg/d)[56]; consequently, they should be considered as a treatment option, especially if SSRIs are not effective.

Obsessive compulsive disorder pharmacology

Despite the frequency of perinatal OCD, surprisingly little research has been done regarding medications during pregnancy and postpartum for this disorder. In contrast to panic disorder and GAD, where lower doses of SSRIs may be effective for anxiety, in OCD, higher doses are generally needed.[39]

Choice of SSRI should be based on prior history of medication efficacy, or if new onset OCD, guided by family history of medication efficacy, and guided by breastfeeding plans. Because sertraline has been shown to have low concentration in breast milk[57] and is an effective treatment of OCD,[58] it could be a reason to choose this medication over fluoxetine in a drug naïve patient, because the extremely high doses of fluoxetine could be associated with greater risk of nursing infant side effects (colic, poor sleep). Fluoxetine has been extensively studied in pregnancy at lower doses than usually used in OCD treatment (20–40 mg/d vs the 60–80 mg/d often needed for OCD) and is an effective treatment of OCD in nonpregnant patients.[58] Clomipramine, a tricycle antidepressant, is also an effective medication for the treatment of OCD, but there is less safety data regarding this medication in pregnancy.[59]

Posttraumatic stress disorder pharmacology

Sertraline and paroxetine are the 2 SSRIs that are approved by Food and Drug Administration for the treatment of PTSD in the general population; venlafaxine is effective as well.[60] No SSRIs have been approved for perinatal PTSD, and in fact no randomized controlled studies have been completed. Nevertheless, for women with perinatal PTSD who do not respond to trauma-focused therapy, treatment with an SSRI (except paroxetine) may be helpful for decreasing PTSD symptoms.

Social anxiety disorder

SSRIs are the psychopharmacologic treatment of choice for social anxiety disorder in the general population, and venlafaxine is used as well.[61] To date, there are no published trials of the effectiveness of these medications in the treatment of social anxiety disorder in pregnant and postpartum women.

Antidepressants During Lactation

SSRIs are compatible with breastfeeding. The most extensively studied medication to date is sertraline, and investigation of mother-infant pairs have consistently shown low levels of medication in mother's breast milk and infant serum after nursing.[58] Other medications with low levels in breast milk are fluvoxamine, paroxetine, and escitalopram. Fluoxetine and citalopram are not contraindicated in breastfeeding, but studies report higher levels in breast milk, but to date no long-term complications of the newborn have been reported.[58] If a patient has found these uniquely effective, it is not recommended that a patient be changed from this medication postpartum or that another medication be trialed. It is important to point out that most SSRI and lactation studies have been completed with patients taking standard doses and not the exceptionally high doses that are used in OCD.

Benzodiazepines During Pregnancy

For patients with severe symptoms of panic disorder or generalized anxiety disorder, temporary use of benzodiazepines may be needed. Benzodiazepines are effective for treatment of panic attacks and symptoms of anxiety, but they should not be considered a long-term treatment plan, because of central nervous system depression and abuse potential as well as continued controversy regarding the association with increased risk of cleft lip and palate if infants are exposed to frequent doses in the first trimester. It is reassuring that most large database studies,[62] recent systematic reviews, and meta-analysis do not report an increased risk of oral cleft defects[63] or congenital malformations.[64] Although others do report an increased risk in case control studies,[65] there is still a low absolute risk of congenital malformation, less than 1%.[65]

The general consensus is that benzodiazepines are not absolutely contraindicated in pregnancy as they were in the past. Short-term use early in the treatment of panic disorder while a patient is tapering onto SSRI may be indicated, but longer-term combined use with SSRIs should be discouraged, because increased risk of congenital anomalies are reported when combined with antidepressants.[66] Patients should be cautioned that daily use of benzodiazepines near to term has also been associated with neonatal withdrawal symptoms, including "floppy baby syndrome,"poor tone, lethargy, hypothermia, and low APGAR scores.[67] Other withdrawal symptoms that may occur include hypertonia, hyperreflexia, and tremors.[68] Benzodiazepines have also been associated with increased rates of ventilator support, cesarean section, and low birth weight.[67]

Benzodiazepines and Lactation

Benzodiazepines are excreted in breast milk, but generally at low concentrations, and they are not contraindicated in breastfeeding. Recent prospective studies have reported low rates of sedation in infants, less than 2%.[69] Benzodiazepines with shorter half-lives are preferred, such as lorazepam. Both diazepam and clonazepam have active metabolites and long half-lives, so they are less preferred for breastfeeding mothers.[58]

Infants should be followed closely for sedation and patients encouraged to discuss the use of this medication with their pediatrician before initiation. When benzodiazepines are combined with other potentially sedating medications, including SSRIs, this increases risk for sedation in infants.[58]

SUMMARY: TREATMENT RECOMMENDATIONS

- Obtain severity of baseline symptoms and continue to monitor treatment effectiveness
- Referral to CBT specialist for intensive CBT and/or mindfulness-based CBT
- For patients with severe symptoms initiation of psychopharmacology in combination with CBT
- In patients with preexisting anxiety disorder, choice of SSRI/SNRI will depend on prior history of efficacy
- For new onset anxiety disorders, sertraline may be a preferred choice because of extensive safety in breastfeeding
- "Start low and go slow" in generalized anxiety and panic disorders: begin patients at half the usual starting dose
- If benzodiazepine is needed while SSRI is being titrated upward, use the lowest possible dose of a short-acting agent such as lorazepam
- Extensive psychoeducation regarding risks and benefits of initiating medication and follow-up/surveillance of infants

REFERENCES

1. Kessler RC, Chiu WT, Demler O, et al. Prevalence, severity, and comorbidity of 12-month DSM-IV disorders in the National Comorbidity Survey Replication. Arch Gen Psychiatry 2005;62(6):617–27.
2. Robertson E, Grace S, Wallington T, et al. Antenatal risk factors for postpartum depression: a synthesis of recent literature. Gen Hosp Psychiatry 2004;26(4): 289–95.
3. Leach LS, Poyser C, Fairweather-Schmidt K. Maternal perinatal anxiety: a review of prevalence and correlates. Clin Psychol 2017;21:4–19.
4. Wenzel A, Stuart S, (Collaborator). Anxiety in childbearing women: diagnosis and treatment. American Psychological Association; 2010.
5. Boyce P, Condon J. Traumatic childbirth and the role of debriefing. In: Raphael B, Wilson JP, editors. Psychological debriefing: theory, practice and evidence. Cambridge (England): Cambridge University Press; 2000. p. 272–80.
6. Torres AR, Prince MJ, Bebbington PE, et al. Obsessive-compulsive disorder: prevalence, comorbidity, impact, and help-seeking in the British National Psychiatric Morbidity Survey of 2000. Am J Psychiatry 2006;163(11):1978–85.
7. Adewuya A, Ola B, Aloba O, et al. Anxiety disorders among Nigerian women in late pregnancy: a controlled study. Arch Womens Ment Health 2006;9:325.
8. Uguz F, Akman C, Kaya N, et al. Postpartum-onset obsessive-compulsive disorder: Incidence, clinical features, and related factors. J Clin Psychiatry 2007;68:132.
9. Wenzel A, Haugen EN, Jackson LC, et al. Anxiety symptoms and disorders at eight weeks postpartum. J Anxiety Disord 2005;19(3):295–311.

10. Abramowitz JS, Foa EB, Franklin ME. Exposure and ritual prevention for obsessive-compulsive disorder: effects of intensive versus twice-weekly sessions. J Consult Clin Psychol 2003;71(2):394–8.
11. Hertzberg T, Wahlbeck K. The impact of pregnancy and puerperium on panic disorder: a review. J Psychosom Obstet Gynaecol 1999;20(2):59–64.
12. Cohen LS, Sichel DA, Dimmock JA, et al. Postpartum course in women with pre-existing panic disorder. J Clin Psychiatry 1994;55(7):289–92.
13. Mota N, Cox BJ, Enns MW, et al. The relationship between mental disorders, quality of life, and pregnancy: findings from a nationally representative sample. J Affect Disord 2008;109:300–4.
14. Ford E, Ayers S, Bradley R. Exploration of a cognitive model to predict posttraumatic stress symptoms following childbirth. J Anxiety Disord 2010;24:353–9.
15. Creedy K, Sochet M, Horsfall J. Childbirth and the development of acute trauma symptoms: incidents and contributing factor. Birth 2000;27(2):105–11.
16. Stuart S, Couser G, Schilder K, et al. Postpartum anxiety and depression: onset and comorbidity in a community sample. J Nerv Ment Dis 1998;186(7):420–4.
17. Accortt EE, Cheadle AC, Dunkel Schetter C. Prenatal depression and adverse birth outcomes: an updated systematic review. Matern Child Health J 2015; 19(6):1306–37.
18. Barnett B, Parker G. Possible determinants, correlates and consequences of high levels of anxiety in primiparous mothers. Psychol Med 1986;16(1):177–85.
19. O'Hara MW, Swain AM. Rates and risk of postpartum depression: a meta-analysis. Int Rev Psychiatry 1996;8:37–54.
20. Van den Bergh BR, Marcoen A. High antenatal maternal anxiety is related to ADHD symptoms, externalizing problems, and anxiety in 8- and 9-year-olds. Child Dev 2004;75:1085–97.
21. O'Connor TG, Heron J, Glover V, the AL SPAC Study Team. Antenatal anxiety predicts child behavioral/emotional problems independently of postnatal depression. J Am Acad Child Adolesc Psychiatry 2002;41(12):1470.
22. Yonkers KA, Smith MV, Forray A, et al. Pregnant women with posttraumatic stress disorder and risk of preterm birth. JAMA Psychiatry 2014;71(8):897–904.
23. Söderquist J, Wijma B, Wijma K. The longitudinal course of post-traumatic stress after childbirth. J Psychosom Obstet Gynaecol 2006;27(2):113–9.
24. Goodman JH, Watson GR, Stubbs B. Anxiety disorders in postpartum women: a systematic review and meta-analysis. J Affective Disord 2016;203:292–331.
25. Bandelow B, Sojka F, Brooks A, et al. Panic disorder during pregnancy and postpartum period. Eur Psychiatry 2006;21(7):495–500.
26. Cerulli C, Chaudron LH, Talbot NI, et al. Co-occurring intimate partner violence and mental diagnoses in perinatal women. J Womens Health (Lachmt) 2011; 20:1797–803.
27. Buist A, Gotman N, Yonkers KA. Generalized anxiety disorder: course and risk factors in pregnancy. J Affect Discord 2011;131(1–3):277–83.
28. Goodman JH, Chenausky KL, Freeman M. Anxiety disorders during pregnancy: a systematic review. J Clin Psych 2014;75(10):e1153–84.
29. Williams K, Koran L. Obsessive-compulsive disorder in pregnancy, the puerperium, and the premenstruum. J Clin Psychiatry 1997;58:330–4.
30. Meltzer Brody S, Larsen JT, Petersen L, et al. Adverse life events increase risk for postpartum psychiatric episodes: a population based epidemiologic study. Depress Anxiety 2018;35(2):160–7.
31. Shaw RJ, Deblois T, Ikuta L, et al. Acute stress disorder among parents of infants in the neonatal intensive care nursery. Psychosomatics 2006;47(3):206–12.

32. Matthey S. Using the Edinburgh postnatal depression scale to screen for anxiety disorders. Depress Anxiety 2008;25:926–31.

33. Spitzer RL, Kroenke K, Williams JB, et al. A brief measure for assessing generalized anxiety disorder: the GAD-7. Arch Intern Med 2006;166(10):1092–7.

34. American Psychiatric Association. APA_DSM5_Severity-Measure-For-Panic-Disorder-Adult.pdf. 2013.

35. Rowa K, Li T, Chan A, et al. Validation of the revised perinatal obsessive-compulsive scale. Preliminary results. F1000Posters 2014;5:460 (poster).

36. Brandes M, Cohen LS, Soares CN. Postpartum onset obsessive-compulsive disorder: diagnosis and management. Arch Womens Ment Health 2004;7:99–110.

37. Quinnell FA, Hynan MT. Convergent and discriminant validity of the perinatal PTSD questionnaire (PPQ): a preliminary study. J Trauma Stress 1999;12:193–9.

38. Foa EB, Riggs DS, Dancu CV, et al. Reliability and validity of a brief instrument for assessing post-traumatic stress disorder. J Trauma Stress 1993;6:459–73.

39. Seibell PJ, Hollander E. Management of obsessive-compulsive disorder. F1000Prime Rep 2014;6:68.

40. Byatt N, Allison J, Levin LL, et al. Enhancing participation in depression care in outpatient perinatal care settings: a systematic review. Obstet Gynecol 2015; 126(5):1048–58.

41. Marchesi C, Ossola P, Amerio A, et al. Clinical management of perinatal anxiety disorders: a systematic review. J Affect Disord 2016;190:543–50.

42. Robinson L, Walker JR, Anderson D. Cognitive-behavioral treatment of panic disorder during pregnancy and lactation. Can J Psychiatry 1992;37:623–6.

43. Austin MP, Acland S, Frilingos M, et al. Brief antenatal cognitive behavior therapy group intervention for the prevention of postnatal depression and anxiety: a randomized controlled trial. Affect Disord 2008;105(1–3):35–44.

44. Koran LM, Hanna GL, Hollander E, et al, American Psychiatric Association. Practice guideline for the treatment of patients with obsessive-compulsive disorder. Am J Psychiatry 2007;164(7 Suppl):5–53.

45. Christian LM, Storch EA. Cognitive behavioral treatment of postpartum onset obsessive compulsive disorder with aggressive obsessions. Clin Case Stud 2009;8(1):72–83.

46. Chelmow D, Halfin VP. Pregnancy complicated by obsessive–compulsive disorder. J Matern Fetal Med 1997;6:31–4.

47. Challacombe FL, Salkovskis PM. Intensive cognitive-behavioural treatment for women with postnatal obsessive-compulsive disorder: a consecutive case series. Behav Res Ther 2011;49:422–6.

48. Wiegartz P, Gyperkoe KL. The pregnancy and postpartum anxiety workbook. Oakland (CA): New Harbinger Publications; 2009.

49. Bastos MH, Bick D, Furura M, et al. Debriefing interventions for the prevention of psychological trauma in women following childbirth. Cochrane Database Syst Rev 2015;(4):CD007194.

50. Ayers S, Bond R, Bertullies S, et al. The aetiology of post-traumatic stress following childbirth: a meta-analysis and theoretical framework. Psychol Med 2016;46:1121–34.

51. De Schepper S, Vercauteren T, Tersago J, et al. Post-traumatic stress disorder after childbirth and the influence of maternity team care during labour and birth: a cohort study. Midwifery 2016;32:87–92.

52. Watts BV, Schnurr PP, Mayo L, et al. Meta-analysis of the efficacy of treatments for posttraumatic stress disorder. J Clin Psychiatry 2013;74(6):541–50.

53. Mayo-Wilson A, Clark Dias K, Mavranezouli P. Psychological and pharmacological interventions for social anxiety disorder in adults: a systematic review and network meta-analysis. Lancet Psychiatry 2014;1(5):368–76.
54. Prady SL, Hanlon I, Fraser LK, et al. A systematic review of maternal antidepressant use in pregnancy and short- and long-term offspring's outcomes. Arch Womens Ment Health 2018;21(2):127–40.
55. Goodman JH. Women's attitudes, preferences, and perceived barriers to treatment for perinatal depression. Birth 2009;36:60–9.
56. Uguz F, Sahingoz M, Gungor B, et al. Low-dose imipramine for treatment of panic disorder during pregnancy: a retrospective chart review. J Clin Psychopharmacol 2014;34:513–5.
57. Kronenfeld N, Berkovitch M, Berlin M, et al. Use of psyschotropic medications in breastfeeding women. Birth Defects Res 2017;109:957–97.
58. Pizarro M, Fontenelle LF, Paravidino DC, et al. An updated review of antidepressants with marked serotonergic effects in obsessive-compulsive disorder. Expert Opin Pharmacother 2014;15(10):1391–401.
59. Uguz F. Pharmacotherapy of obsessive compulsive disorder during pregnancy: a clinical approach. Rev Bras Psiquiatr 2015;37(4):334–42.
60. Bernardy NC, Friedman MJ. Pharmacologic management of PTSD. Curr Opin Psychol 2017;14:116–21.
61. Blanco C, Bragdon LB, Liebowitz MR, et al. The evidence-based pharmacotherapy of social anxiety disorder. Int J Neuropsychopharmacol 2013;16(1):235–49.
62. Wikner BN, Stiller CO, Bergman U, et al. Use of benzodiazepines and benzodiazepine receptor agonists during pregnancy: neonatal outcome and congenital malformations. Pharmacoepidemiol Drug Saf 2007;16(11):1203–10.
63. Okun ML, Ebert R, Saini B. A review of sleep-promoting medications used in pregnancy. Am J Obstet Gynecol 2015;212(4):428–41.
64. Dolovich LR, Addis A, Vaillancourt JM, et al. Benzodiazepine use in pregnancy and major malformations or oral cleft: meta-analysis of cohort and case–control studies. BMJ 1998;317:839–43.
65. Enato E, Koren G, Moretti M. The fetal safety of benzodiazepines: update meta-analysis. J Obstet Gynaecol Can 2011;33(1):46–8.
66. Oberlander TF, Aghajanian J, Hertzman C, et al. Major congenital malformations following prenatal exposure to serotonin reuptake inhibitors and benzodiazepines using population-based health data. Birth Defects Res B Dev Reprod Toxicol 2008;83(1):68–76.
67. Yonkers KA, Gilstad-Hayden K, Forray A, et al. Association of panic disorder, generalized anxiety disorder, and benzodiazepine treatment during pregnancy with risk of adverse birth outcomes. JAMA Psychiatry 2017;74(11):1145–52.
68. Iqbal MM, Ryals T, Sobhan T. Effects of commonly used benzodiazepines on the fetus, the neonate, and the nursing infant. Psychiatr Serv 2002;53:39–49.
69. Kelly LE, Poon S, Madadi P, et al. Neonatal benzodiazepines exposure during breastfeeding. J Pediatr 2012;161(3):448–51.

Perinatal Sleep Problems
Causes, Complications, and Management

Allison K. Wilkerson, PhD*, Thomas W. Uhde, MD

KEYWORDS

• Sleep • Insomnia • Pregnancy • Peripartum • Postpartum

KEY POINTS

• Changes in sleep duration and sleep fragmentation during the perinatal period are well-documented using subjective and objective measures.
• Sleep deficiency indicating the need for more targeted sleep intervention is caused by sleep disorders, physiologic changes, or alterations in mood.
• Evidence-based behavioral and pharmacologic interventions are used effectively in this population.

Changes in sleep occur throughout pregnancy and the postpartum period, with sleep disturbance typically increasing in the later months of gestation and first few postpartum weeks. The course and nature of sleep disturbance in the perinatal period has been well-documented via self-report measures and objective measures, such as actigraphy (a wearable device designed to detect sleep and wake) and polysomnography (PSG; overnight sleep study). A growing body of literature has shown that these changes in sleep patterns, historically seen as normal and tolerable, have the potential to serve as a catalyst for negative physical and mental health consequences. Thus improving sleep can serve as a modifiable risk factor for intervention throughout this important period of adulthood.[1] This is particularly pertinent to women today because the number of women working throughout pregnancy and in early postpartum has grown exponentially in recent years,[2] limiting many of the more obvious options for treating perinatal sleep problems, such as sleeping in or scheduling naps.

The present review provides a synopsis of subjective and objective changes in sleep patterns during the perinatal period. Causes and complicating factors that increase the risk for problematic sleep deficiency and its consequences are then summarized, and potential management strategies are discussed.

Disclosure Statement: The authors have no commercial or financial conflicts of interest to disclose.
Department of Psychiatry and Behavioral Sciences, Medical University of South Carolina, 67 President Street, MSC 861, Charleston, SC 29425, USA
* Corresponding author.
E-mail address: wilkersa@musc.edu

Obstet Gynecol Clin N Am 45 (2018) 483–494
https://doi.org/10.1016/j.ogc.2018.04.003   obgyn.theclinics.com

SUBJECTIVE SLEEP

Several different self-report methodologies have been used to explore perceived changes in sleep during the perinatal period, including single-item questions, structured interviews, questionnaires assessing multiple domains of sleep, and daily sleep diaries. Most studies have used the latter 2 options because they provide comprehensive information without the burden of time and resources to train and schedule staff to conduct interviews.

Questionnaires

Multiple self-report questionnaires have found a similar pattern of sleep changes throughout pregnancy and the early postpartum period. Two of the most common questionnaires used have been the General Sleep Disturbance Scale (GSDS)[3] and the Pittsburgh Sleep Quality Index (PSQI).[4]

The GSDS was initially designed for women and has often been used in perinatal populations.[5,6] This 21-item questionnaire assesses perception of sleep during the previous week, covering a variety of general sleep issues, including difficulty initiating sleep, waking up during sleep, quality of sleep, daytime sleepiness, and substance use. All questions are answered on a Likert scale from 0 to 7 and added together resulting in a total score between 0 and 147, with greater than 43 as a cutoff for poor sleepers. Several studies have found mean scores of women to be greater than 43 in the third trimester and first postpartum month, nearing or dropping below the cutoff around the third postpartum month.[6–10]

The PSQI has also been well-validated in this population.[11] This 19-item questionnaire assesses perception of sleep over the previous month, covering the domains of sleep quality, sleep latency, sleep duration, sleep efficiency, sleep disturbances, use of sleep medications, and subsequent daytime dysfunction. Each domain is scored separately and the domains are added together to produce a global score between 0 and 21, with a score greater than 5 as a cutoff distinguishing poor sleepers from good sleepers. Several studies have used the PSQI to examine sleep earlier in pregnancy. Those studies that have observed women longitudinally reported a gradual increase in score (indicating worsening sleep) from early to late pregnancy, with a sharp increase in the days and weeks immediately following birth and a slow decline through the postpartum months (indicating a return toward good sleep).[12–18] Moreover, in most of the studies that have administered the PSQI at any point during this time period, mean scores at every time point from first trimester through early postpartum exceeded the cutoff score of 5, indicating poor sleep throughout this period.[12,14–17,19–21] The one exception to this was a study by Okun and colleagues, who found mean scores of 4.9 and 4.5 in the first and second trimester, respectively. This is perhaps because of a small sample size ($n = 19$) of primarily well-educated, married, working women with resources to help optimize sleep, although even this group neared the cutoff score.

Sleep Diaries

The purpose of a sleep diary is to prospectively assess daily sleep over a given period of time by having an individual complete several questions regarding the previous day and night, preferably on awakening, to help ensure within subject validity and consistency of data collection across subjects. Although there are several variations of sleep diaries in circulation, most provide the same standard sleep parameters, including total sleep time (TST) during the previous night and/or the previous 24 hours, sleep onset latency (SOL, amount of time taken to fall asleep), and wake after sleep onset (WASO, amount of time awake throughout the night).[22] Sleep diaries have been used far less than questionnaires in this population but reveal findings consistent with that of the questionnaires. One study administered sleep diaries in the first, second, and third trimester[13]; one study in third trimester only[23]; one study in the third trimester and the first and third postpartum months[24]; and one study in the second month.[25] Surprisingly, TST, a measure of sleep duration, remained consistent across all trimesters and postpartum months, averaging 7 to 8 hours per night. SOL also showed little variability, with averages in each sample ranging from 10 to 25 minutes at all time points. However, WASO, a measure of sleep fragmentation, changed markedly over the course of pregnancy, increasing from approximately 30 minutes in the first and second trimester to 35 to 60 minutes in the third trimester, 2 hours in the first postpartum month, and declining to approximately 90 minutes and 60 minutes in the second and third month, respectively. Given none of these studies observed the same group from first trimester to the postpartum months it is difficult to draw definitive conclusions regarding the expected parameters for these variables in the general perinatal population because each study had a different sample with different demographics. However, taken together they indicate self-reported sleep fragmentation (WASO), than sleep duration (TST), that is, the hallmark of sleep changes during this period.

OBJECTIVE SLEEP
Actigraphy

Given the challenges of transitioning a new baby into the family and home environment, actigraphy has often been used as a noninvasive method to objectively measure sleep and activity levels to accurately collect sleep parameters while not greatly increasing participant burden. Multiple studies have used actigraphy to longitudinally understand sleep duration and sleep fragmentation via TST and WASO, beginning in the second or third trimester. Similar to sleep diaries, most studies had mean TST of 7 to 8 hours during pregnancy.[6,15,16,26–28] However, unlike sleep diaries, these studies showed a drop in TST from late pregnancy to the first postpartum month, with averages ranging between 5.5 to 7 hours per night and increasing gradually over the following months. Similar to sleep diaries, most studies showed a significant increase in WASO from late pregnancy to the first month postpartum, with WASO in the third trimester averaging 50 to 80 minutes, increasing to 1.5 to 2.5 hours in the first postpartum month, and gradually decreasing over subsequent weeks and months.[6,15,16,26]

Two studies have shown slight differences to these findings. One study found a less severe increase in WASO in late pregnancy and early postpartum. However, these findings were based on a full 24-hour cycle that included naps, a sleep period much less likely to be associated with awakenings compared with typical nocturnal sleep.[27] The second found TST to be between 7.5 and 8.5 at third trimester and the first 3 postpartum months. This same study found WASO to be nearly double that of all other studies at all time points.[10] The reason for this discrepancy is also likely related to methodological sources of variance but warrants further investigation.

Taken together, these investigations show a consistent pattern of worsening sleep from late pregnancy through most of the first postpartum period, as evidenced by decreased TST and/or increased WASO using objective actigraphy methodology.

Polysomnography

PSG is considered the "gold standard" of sleep assessment, although it requires significant participant burden (eg, multiple electrodes attached, arrangement of nocturnal childcare, and often sleeping away from home if an in-home study cannot be arranged) and is subsequently the least used methodology in studies of sleep in perinatal women. Studies using PSGs in this population indicate sleep diaries and actigraphy may be overestimating sleep parameters. Although the overall pattern of change in sleep disturbance over this time period is similar, the average TST and WASO are somewhat different using PSG versus actigraphy or self-reported sleep diaries. In one study women underwent PSG during the last month of pregnancy and at 3 times during postpartum (the first, third, and sixth weeks).[29] They found TST to be between 5 to 6 hours at every time point, with WASO approximately 20 minutes in third trimester increasing to 70 to 80 minutes during the postpartum time points. Another study observed women before pregnancy, conducting PSGs in their homes for 2 nights during prepregnancy, once each trimester, and during the first and third months postpartum.[30] The investigators found TST at all time points to average 6 to 7.5 hours per night, with the lowest average in the first postpartum month. WASO ranged from 25 to 50 minutes in pregnancy with an increase to approximately 70 minutes in the first postpartum month.

In summary, subjective and objective measures of quantitative sleep parameters indicate consistent sleep duration throughout pregnancy with a gradual increase in sleep fragmentation from first trimester through third trimester. Women subjectively report that sleep duration remains consistent during the transition from pregnancy to postpartum, although objective measures indicate a decrease in sleep duration after the birth of the child, increasing over the subsequent weeks and months. Both subjective and objective measures reveal a significant increase in sleep fragmentation following the birth, increasing over the subsequent months. Despite some of these sleep parameters resembling characteristics of healthy, normal sleep (eg, sleep duration of 7 hours per night),[31] women endorse poor overall sleep throughout the pregnancy and postpartum period on questionnaires that assess multiple domains of sleep, such as sleep quality and daytime dysfunction as a result of poor sleep.

SLEEP DEFICIENCY

The point at which these sleep changes become problematic is difficult to identify as the terminology and definitions that describe sleep disturbance vary throughout the literature. The term "sleep deficiency" was introduced by the National Center for Sleep Disorders Research (NCSDR) in 2011 as a way to categorize and understand problematic sleep patterns that are associated with increased disease risk.[32] Buxton and colleagues[33] suggested sleep deficiency can be best operationally defined through 3 sleep variables:

1. Insomnia symptoms
2. Short sleep duration
3. Sleep insufficiency (feeling unrested on awakening)

Okun and colleagues[34] adapted and further refined this definition for perinatal populations, specifically the following:

1. Insomnia symptoms were defined as self-reported difficulty falling or staying asleep with subsequent daytime dysfunction,
2. Short sleep duration was defined as less than 7 hours via self-reported sleep diary and less than 6 hours via actigraphy, and
3. Sleep insufficiency was defined as self-reported experience of unrefreshing sleep on a frequent basis.

Although there is substantial overlap among the 3 sleep deficiency variables, it is important to highlight they can also be different. For example, someone who does not experience the insomnia symptoms of difficulty falling or staying asleep (variable 1) but only allows herself to sleep 5 to 6 hours because of other obligations or personal preference would still be considered sleep-deficient due to the short sleep duration (variable 2). Similarly, someone who spends at least 8 hours sleeping with a perception of only minor interruptions but wakes up feeling unrested is not experiencing insomnia symptoms (variable 1) or short sleep duration (variable 2) but is experiencing insufficient sleep (variable 3) and may be suffering an underlying sleep disorder, such as sleep apnea. See **Table 1** for a comparison of expected perinatal sleep changes versus sleep changes indicating sleep deficiency and subsequent targeted intervention.

Indeed, these 3 factors are important in the perinatal period as insomnia symptoms have been linked to higher blood pressure and body mass index as well as peripartum depression.[8,35] Short sleep duration has been linked to spontaneous preterm delivery, longer delivery times, and more pain during labor, as well as increased likelihood of gestational diabetes, hypertension, preeclampsia, caesarean section, peripartum depression, and low infant birth weight.[7,13,36,37] Insufficient sleep, such as that linked with breathing-related sleep disorders or the prolonged sleep fragmentation that occurs in the early postpartum weeks, has been linked to hypertensive disorders, gestational diabetes, and declining cognitive performance.[38,39]

Causes and Complicating Factors in Pregnancy

The literature to date indicates that some demographic characteristics are risk factors for sleep deficiency. Women who are employed or older than 30 years have been found to be more likely to have short sleep duration.[18,40] Women older than 35 years and those who are African American or of Hispanic ethnoracial status have been found to be more likely to have poor sleep via the PSQI.[18] Evidence for the relationship between parity and sleep deficiency is minimal, although 2 studies using objective measures suggest that nullipara experience more sleep deficiency, primarily shorter sleep duration, than multipara during pregnancy and early postpartum.[27,30]

Table 1
Expected sleep changes compared with changes indicating sleep deficiency in the perinatal period

Common Sleep Changes in Perinatal Period Requiring Routing Management	Indicators of Sleep Deficiency That May Require Targeted Treatment Intervention
• Insomnia symptoms: intermittent difficulty falling or staying asleep, although not enough to be a major contributor to daytime disturbance • Decreased sleep duration: a gradual decline in total sleep time due to increased sleep fragmentation in pregnancy and the postpartum period, but generally able to maintain consistent duration by going to bed early, sleeping in, or napping • Sleep insufficiency: intermittent experience of feeling nonrefreshed on awakening, although not enough to be a major contributor to daytime disturbance	• Insomnia symptoms: self-reported difficulty falling or staying asleep at least 3 times per week with subsequent daytime disturbance • Decreased sleep duration: <7 h of self-reported sleep per night or <6 h of sleep per night measured using actigraphy • Sleep insufficiency: feeling nonrested on awakening (despite adequate sleep environment and time to sleep) almost every night with subsequent daytime disturbance; often associated with OSA, RLS

Sleep disorders are perhaps the most obvious cause of sleep deficiency in pregnancy. Three of the most common sleep disorders found in pregnancy are insomnia, breathing-related sleep disorders, and restless leg syndrome (RLS).[41] Insomnia is defined as difficulty initiating or maintaining sleep with subsequent impairment in daytime functioning, at least 3 times per week for at least 3 months.[42] Prevalence of insomnia throughout all 3 trimesters and the early postpartum period range from 45%–70%, which is significantly higher than the general population (10%–15%).[43–46]

The primary breathing-related sleep disorder in pregnancy is obstructive sleep apnea (OSA), which is characterized by nocturnal breathing disturbances (ie, snoring, snorting/gasping, and/or breathing pauses during sleep) and daytime sleepiness, fatigue, or unrefreshing sleep; a diagnosis must be confirmed via PSG.[42] Prevalence rates in pregnancy are unclear, likely because the role of OSA in pregnancy is complicated, because some characteristics of pregnancy are protective against breathing-related sleep problems, such as increased respiratory drive and preference for lateral sleeping (as opposed to supine, which is more likely to restrict the airway), whereas other characteristics of pregnancy are well-known predisposing factors of breathing-related sleep problems, including nasal congestion and reduced functional residual capacity.[38,41]

RLS is defined as an uncomfortable sensation in the legs characterized by an urge to move that worsens during periods of rest/inactivity and/or in the evening; it is relieved by movement, occurs at least 3 times per week for at least 3 months, and results in daytime impairment.[42] Prevalence of RLS increases markedly during pregnancy, steadily increasing from first through third trimesters and virtually dissipates following delivery.[18,40,47,48] Given these symptoms worsen at night, many women report difficulty falling and staying sleeping because of these irritating and painful sensations. The increase in RLS symptoms during pregnancy have been attributed to low levels of iron and high levels of estradiol, although a few recent studies have failed to support these conclusions.[38]

Physical and hormonal changes also play a role in sleep deficiency during pregnancy. Increasing discomfort due to weight gain and changing body shape can be accompanied by several complaints, including nausea, need to urinate, headaches, fetal movement, joint pain, difficulty finding a comfortable position, and muscle cramping.[45,49] There is a large increase in progesterone, estradiol, estriol, and prolactin over the course of pregnancy, which is thought to make women sleepier, indicating sleep insufficiency; however, varying methodologies and operational definitions across studies as well as lack of longitudinal designs using objective measures of sleep and sleepiness related to biomarkers makes it difficult to draw definitive conclusions.[50]

The positive relationship between poor sleep and depression during pregnancy has been extensively studied and systematically reviewed.[51,52] In summary, this relationship seems to be reciprocal throughout the gestational period. Perception of sleep deficiency via questionnaires and sleep diaries is strongly correlated with depressive symptomatology. Objective measures have less support, although changes in fragmentation seem to be more important than changes in sleep duration.

Management in Pregnancy

Nonpharmacologic treatment strategies are typically used as first-line treatments for sleep deficiency in pregnancy although there is a paucity of research exploring the efficacy of evidence-based behavioral interventions adapted for this population (**Table 2**). A small pilot study (n = 26) examining massage therapy for 20 minutes, twice per week for 5 weeks, beginning in the second trimester improved several

Table 2
Summary of treatment options

Presenting Sleep Complaint	Approach	Treatment

Insomnia and/or short sleep duration	Confirm frequency of disturbance and severity of related impairment
	Identify possible related anxiety/worry
	Identify prior effective medications
		1. Encourage sleep hygiene/healthy sleep habits
		2. CBTI adapted for pregnancy
		3. Pharmacology, initiate with lowest recommended dose (eg, zolpidem, 5 mg; alprazolam, .25 mg)
		  a. Moderate to severe: hypnotic
		  b. Severe insomnia (particularly if comorbid anxiety): benzodiazepine

OSA	Confirm with PSG	1. CPAP 2. Recommend daily exercise (if related to excessive weight gain)
RLS	Check iron level	1. Iron supplement if <50 mcg/dl 2. Recommend daily exercise 3. CBTI adapted for RLS

Abbreviations: CBTI, cognitive behavioral therapy for insomnia; CPAP, continuous positive airway pressure.

aspects of sleep quality via a 15-item measure consisting of visual analog scales.[53] Another small study (*n* = 15) examining mindful yoga on sleep in pregnant women in their second or third trimester found attending a weekly class for 7 weeks reduced number of awakenings during the night, time awake at night, and perceived sleep disturbance.[54] Most recently, another pilot study (*n* = 13) delivered 5 weeks of cognitive behavioral therapy for insomnia (CBTI), the most effective nonpharmacologic insomnia treatment in the general population, to women in their second trimester with insomnia.[55] Consistent with CBTI for the general population, each 90 minutes session in this trial covered a sleep topic: introduction to sleep diaries, psychoeducation about sleep, stimulus control (using the bed only for sleep and sex), modifying thoughts to promote positive and functional beliefs about sleep, and relapse prevention. Women showed significant improvement on multiple well-validated sleep questionnaires as well as several sleep parameters measured via sleep diaries and actigraphy.

For sleep complaints related to OSA and RLS there are different management approaches. There is little treatment literature exploring continuous positive airway pressure (CPAP) and other treatment options for sleep apnea and other breathing-related sleep problems in this population. To date, the primary suggestions are to follow the guidelines created for the nonpregnant populations, although the literature on this is mixed.[38] One of the most common treatments for RLS in this population is iron supplements, although this is based on a few studies with small sample sizes.[47,56] There is sufficient evidence for behavioral interventions for RLS, which has been reviewed thoroughly by Pigeon and colleagues.[56] In summary, a sleep hygiene handout with instructions is likely ineffective (particularly as pregnant women are already practicing the most common sleep hygiene suggestions, including avoiding alcohol, tobacco, and caffeine excess); however, a more thorough, interactive discussion of techniques of CBTI adapted for RLS has been shown to have an effect similar to that of medications. Exercise has also been explored as an alternative option, because one hypothesis is that RLS is a result of inactivity, although these results are mixed.

Medication to improve sleep deficiency in pregnancy is considered when nonpharmacologic approaches have failed and/or the sleep-related impairments are greater than the side effects and risks associated with medication.[38] Options for medication often depend on past treatment of sleep problems and current severity.[57] If sleep deficiency is longstanding and medications have worked in the past, these can often be used again in pregnancy if side effects are tolerable and risks are low. Otherwise, for moderate to severe insomnia, hypnotic benzodiazepine receptor antagonists (eg, zolpidem) are most commonly prescribed for use as needed. For more severe insomnia, particularly if there is associated anxiety, benzodiazepines (eg, alprazolam) may be considered for use as needed. There is often a reluctance of pregnant women to ask for or providers to prescribe these medications because of fear of teratogenic effects. However, research on the use of such medications and subsequent infant and maternal outcomes has been recently reviewed in detail, revealing there has been no connection made between these drugs and infant congenital malformations.[38,58] Further, across multiple studies these drugs had no connection with any negative pregnancy outcome, aside from one Taiwanese study of more than 15,000 women that found women taking zolpidem were more likely to have preterm birth, cesarean sections, or infants with low birth weight.

Causes and Complicating Factors in Postpartum

The most obvious addition to the causes of sleep deficiency in the postpartum period compared with pregnancy is the experience of and recovery from labor followed by the nocturnal awakenings of an infant. Sleep is drastically altered during this time. Using actigraphy, Beebe and Lee found that sleep duration decreased in the 5 days before labor, with less than 6 hours sleep the night before delivery.[59] Lee and colleagues[60] also used actigraphy to follow women during the first postpartum week and found that those with cesarean birth had 4 hours of total sleep time, whereas those with vaginal birth averaged 6.5 hours.

Regarding sleep disorders that contribute to sleep deficiency, as previously discussed, the rates of sleep-related breathing problems and RLS decrease markedly following birth. However, a high prevalence of insomnia persists.

There is also a dramatic shift in hormones contributing to changes in sleep during this time. There is a sharp decline in progesterone and estrogen immediately following birth, although the contribution of this change to sleep differences is difficult to tell as it is confounded by the constant sleep interruptions of healing and infant needs.[30,50,61] Further into the postpartum period it has been suggested that increased prolactin increases sleepiness and deep, restorative sleep, particularly in healthy, breastfeeding mothers.

Similar to pregnancy, the relationship between poor sleep and depression during the postpartum period has been extensively studied and recently reviewed.[62,63] Data synthesis of 13 studies found a strong correlation between depressive symptoms and subjective and objective measures of sleep.[62] Again, sleep fragmentation plays an important role, because authors of several studies have hypothesized that the development of depression is largely driven by fatigue and related consequences that are a result of the marked increase in sleep fragmentation that comes with caring for an infant throughout the night.[63–65]

Management in Postpartum

Nonpharmacalogic interventions for sleep have received increased attention in recent years. One large, multisite randomized controlled trial (n = 246) found a 45 to 60 minute information session about sleep and sleep hygiene with a nurse during the hospital stay with 3 brief follow-up calls over the course of 4 weeks did not affect any sleep variables compared with controls who were provided with usual care.[66] Adding another component to this, another large randomized controlled trial (n = 240) met with women in the last trimester and provided them with a bassinet for infant proximity, a noise machine for noise attenuation, and a night light for low lighting, as well as a laminated card describing the importance of these factors.[9] A control group was provided with a brief, in-person informational session about eating habits and a healthy diet. Follow-ups were conducted in the first, second, and third postpartum month. Actigraphy results indicate that the intervention did not improve the sleep parameters of socioeconomically advantaged women but did improve sleep among their less advantaged counterparts compared with controls. Finally, a recent study conducted a more in depth intervention of 5 weeks of CBTI in a small sample of women with postpartum depression (n = 12). Similar to the CBTI intervention in pregnancy study described earlier, these investigators found significant improvements in multiple sleep and fatigue questionnaires as well as several sleep diary variables.[67] Hesitation to improve sleep via medication often persist from pregnancy into the postpartum because of concerns related to breastfeeding; however, occasional benzodiazepine use and short-term use of zolpidem are acceptable according to the American Academy of Pediatrics.[38,68]

REFERENCES

1. Sharkey KM. Time to treat problematic sleep disturbance in perinatal women. Behav Sleep Med 2013;11(4):308–10.
2. Laughlin LL. Maternity leave and employment patterns of first-time mothers: 1961-2008. Washington, DC: US Department of Commerce, Economics and Statistics Administration, US Census Bureau; 2011.
3. Lee KA. Self-reported sleep disturbances in employed women. Sleep 1992;15(6): 493–8.
4. Buysse DJ, Reynolds CF, Monk TH, et al. The Pittsburgh sleep quality index: a new instrument for psychiatric practice and research. Psychiatry Res 1989;28:193–213.
5. Goyal D, Gay C, Lee K. Fragmented maternal sleep is more strongly correlated with depressive symptoms than infant temperament at three months postpartum. Arch Womens Ment Health 2009;12(4):229–37.
6. Gay CL, Lee KA, Lee S-Y. Sleep patterns and fatigue in new mothers and fathers. Biol Res Nurs 2004;5(4):311–8.
7. Lee KA, Gay CL. Sleep in late pregnancy predicts length of labor and type of delivery. Am J Obstet Gynecol 2004;191(6):2041–6.
8. Goyal D, Gay CL, Lee KA. Patterns of sleep disruption and depressive symptoms in new mothers. J Perinat Neonatal Nurs 2007;21(2):6.
9. Lee KA, Gay CL. Can modifications to the bedroom environment improve the sleep of new parents? Two randomized controlled trials. Res Nurs Health 2011; 34(1):7–19.
10. Park EM, Meltzer-Brody S, Stickgold R. Poor sleep maintenance and subjective sleep quality are associated with postpartum maternal depression symptom severity. Arch Womens Ment Health 2013;16(6):539–47.
11. Jomeen J, Martin CR. Assessment and relationship of sleep quality to depression in early pregnancy. J Reprod Infant Psychol 2007;25(1):87–99.
12. Kamysheva E, Skouteris H, Wertheim EH, et al. A prospective investigation of the relationships among sleep quality, physical symptoms, and depressive symptoms during pregnancy. J Affect Disord 2010;123(1–3):317–20.

13. Okun ML, Hall M, Coussons-Read ME. Sleep disturbances increase interleukin-6 production during pregnancy: implications for pregnancy complications. Reprod Sci 2007;14(6):560–7.
14. Skouteris H, Germano C, Wertheim EH, et al. Sleep quality and depression during pregnancy: a prospective study. J Sleep Res 2008;17(2):217–20.
15. Coo S, Milgrom J, Trinder J. Mood and objective and subjective measures of sleep during late pregnancy and the postpartum period. Behav Sleep Med 2014;12(4):317–30.
16. Bei B, Milgrom J, Ericksen J, et al. Subjective perception of sleep, but not its objective quality, is associated with immediate postpartum mood disturbances in healthy women. Sleep 2010;33(4):7.
17. Okun ML, Luther J, Prather AA, et al. Changes in sleep quality, but not hormones predict time to postpartum depression recurrence. J Affect Disord 2011;130(3): 378–84.
18. Facco FL, Kramer J, Ho KH, et al. Sleep disturbances in pregnancy. Obstet Gynecol 2010;115(1):6.
19. Dørheim SK, Bondevik GT, Eberhard-Gran M, et al. Sleep and depression in postpartum women: a population-based study. Sleep 2009;32(7):9.
20. Huang C, Carter PA, Jong-Long G. A comparison of sleep and daytime sleepiness in depressed and non-depressed mothers during the early postpartum period. J Nurs Res 2004;12(4):8.
21. Ko SH, Chang SC, Chen CH. A comparative study of sleep quality between pregnant and nonpregnant Taiwanese women. J Nurs Scholarsh 2010;42(1): 23–30.
22. Carney CE, Buysse DJ, Ancoli-Israel S, et al. The consensus sleep diary: standardizing prospective sleep self-monitoring. Sleep 2012;35(2):287–302.
23. Greenwood KM, Hazendonk KM. Self-reported sleep during the third trimester of pregnancy. Behav Sleep Med 2004;2(4):191–204.
24. Wolfson AR, Carskadon MA. Understanding adolescents' sleep patterns and school performance: a critical appraisal. Sleep Med Rev 2003;7(6):491–506.
25. Dorheim SK, Bondevik GT, Eberhard-Gran M, et al. Subjective and objective sleep among depressed and non-depressed postnatal women. Acta Psychiatr Scand 2009;119(2):128–36.
26. Matsumoto K, Shinkoda H, Kang MJ, et al. Longitudinal study of mothers' sleep-wake behaviors and circadian time patterns from late pregnancy to postpartum - monitoring of wrist actigraphy and sleep logs. Biol Rhythm Res 2003; 34(3):14.
27. Signal TL, Gander PH, Sangalli MR, et al. Sleep duration and quality in healthy nulliparous and multiparous women across pregnancy and post-partum. Aust N Z J Obstet Gynaecol 2007;47(1):16–22.
28. Wulff K, Siegmund R. Circadian and ultradian time patterns in human behaviour: part 1: activity monitoring of families from prepartum to postpartum. Biol Rhythm Res 2000;31(5):581–602.
29. Nishihara KH, Horiuchi S. Changes in sleep patterns of young women from later pregnancy to postpartum: relationships to their infants' movements. Percept Mot Skills 1998;87:14.
30. Lee KA, Zaffke ME, McEnany G. Parity and sleep patterns during and after pregnancy. Obstet Gynecol 2000;95(1):5.
31. Hirshkowitz M, Whiton K, Albert SM, et al. National Sleep Foundation's sleep time duration recommendations: methodology and results summary. Sleep Health 2015;1(1):40–3.

32. Research NCoSD. National Institutes of Health sleep disorders research plan. Bethesda (MD): National Institutes of Health; 2011.
33. Buxton OM, Karen Hopcia N, Sembajwe G, et al. Relationship of sleep deficiency to perceived pain and functional limitations in hospital patient care workers. J Occup Environ Med 2012;54(7):851.
34. Okun ML, Kline CE, Roberts JM, et al. Prevalence of sleep deficiency in early gestation and its associations with stress and depressive symptoms. J Womens Health (Larchmt) 2013;22(12):1028–37.
35. Haney A, Buysse DJ, Rosario BL, et al. Sleep disturbance and cardiometabolic risk factors in early pregnancy: a preliminary study. Sleep Med 2014;15(4):444–50.
36. Chang JJ, Pien GW, Duntley SP, et al. Sleep deprivation during pregnancy and maternal and fetal outcomes: is there a relationship? Sleep Med Rev 2010;14(2):107–14.
37. Palagini L, Gemignani A, Banti S, et al. Chronic sleep loss during pregnancy as a determinant of stress: impact on pregnancy outcome. Sleep Med 2014;15(8):853–9.
38. Oyiengo D, Louis M, Hott B, et al. Sleep disorders in pregnancy. Clin Chest Med 2014;35(3):571–87.
39. Insana SP, Williams KB, Montgomery-Downs HE. Sleep disturbance and neurobehavioral performance among postpartum women. Sleep 2013;36(1):73–81.
40. Hedman C, Pohjasvaara T, Tolonen U, et al. Effects of pregnancy on mothers' sleep. Sleep Med 2002;3(1):37–42.
41. Pien GW, Schwab RJ. Sleep disorders during pregnancy. Sleep 2004;27(7):12.
42. American Psychiatric Association. Diagnostic and statistical manual of mental disorders. 5th edition. Washington, DC: American Psychiatric Publishing; 2013.
43. Lopes EA, Carvalho LB, Seguro PB, et al. Sleep disorders in pregnancy. Arq Neuropsiquiatr 2004;62(2A):217–21.
44. Dorheim SK, Bjorvatn B, Eberhard-Gran M. Insomnia and depressive symptoms in late pregnancy: a population-based study. Behav Sleep Med 2012;10(3):152–66.
45. Mindell JA, Cook RA, Nikolovski J. Sleep patterns and sleep disturbances across pregnancy. Sleep Med 2015;16(4):483–8.
46. Sivertsen B, Eberhard-Gran M, Hysing M, et al. Trajectories of maternal sleep problems before and after childbirth: a longitudinal population-based study. BMC Pregnancy Childbirth 2015;15(1):129.
47. Lee KA, Zaffke ME, Baratte-Beebe K. Restless legs syndrome and sleep disturbance during pregnancy: the role of folate and iron. J Womens Health Gend Based Med 2001;10(4):335–41.
48. Manconi M, Govoni V, De Vito A, et al. Restless legs syndrome and pregnancy. Neurology 2004;63(6):1065–9.
49. Baratte-Beebe KR, Lee K. Sources of midsleep awakenings in childbearing women. Clin Nurs Res 1999;8(4):386–97.
50. Parry BL, Martínez LF, Maurer EL, et al. Sleep, rhythms and women's mood. Part I. menstrual cycle, pregnancy and postpartum. Sleep Med Rev 2006;10(2):129–44.
51. Ross LE, Murray BJ, Steiner M. Sleep and perinatal mood disorders: a critical review. J Psychiatry Neurosci 2005;30(4):9.
52. Bei B, Coo S, Trinder J. Sleep, and mood during pregnancy and the postpartum period. Sleep Med Clin 2015;10(1):25–33.
53. Field T, Hernandez-Reif M, Hart S, et al. Pregnant women benefit from massage therapy. J Psychosom Obstet Gynecol 1999;20(1):31–8.

54. Beddoe AE, Lee KA, Weiss SJ, et al. Effects of mindful yoga on sleep in pregnant women: a pilot study. Biol Res Nurs 2010;11(4):363–70.
55. Tomfohr-Madsen LM, Clayborne ZM, Rouleau CR, et al. Sleeping for two: an open-pilot study of cognitive behavioral therapy for insomnia in pregnancy. Behav Sleep Med 2017;15(5):377–93.
56. Pigeon WR, Yurcheshen M. Behavioral sleep medicine interventions for restless legs syndrome and periodic limb movement disorder. Sleep Med Clin 2009; 4(4):487–94.
57. Hashmi AM, Bhatia SK, Bhatia SK, et al. Insomnia during pregnancy: diagnosis and rational interventions. Pak J Med Sci 2016;32(4):1030.
58. Okun ML, Ebert R, Saini B. A review of sleep-promoting medications used in pregnancy. Am J Obstet Gynecol 2015;212(4):428–41.
59. Beebe KR, Lee KA. Sleep disturbance in late pregnancy and early labor. J Perinat Neonatal Nurs 2007;21(2):103–8.
60. Lee S-Y, Lee KA. Early postpartum sleep and fatigue for mothers after cesarean delivery compared with vaginal delivery: an exploratory study. J Perinat Neonatal Nurs 2007;21(2):109–13.
61. Lee KA, McEnany G, Zaffke MEREM. Sleep and mood state in childbearing women: sleepy or weepy? Sleep 2000;23(7):9.
62. Bhati S, Richards K. A systematic review of the relationship between postpartum sleep disturbance and postpartum depression. J Obstet Gynecol Neonatal Nurs 2015;44(3):350–7.
63. Hunter LP, Rychnovsky JD, Yount SM. A selective review of maternal sleep characteristics in the postpartum period. J Obstet Gynecol Neonatal Nurs 2009;38(1): 60–8.
64. Armitage R, Flynn H, Hoffmann R, et al. Early developmental changes in sleep in infants: the impact of maternal depression. Sleep 2009;32(5):693–6.
65. Dennis CL, Ross L. Relationships among infant sleep patterns, maternal fatigue, and development of depressive symptomatology. Birth 2005;32(3):187–93.
66. Stremler R, Hodnett E, Kenton L, et al. Effect of behavioural-educational intervention on sleep for primiparous women and their infants in early postpartum: multisite randomised controlled trial. BMJ 2013;346:f1164.
67. Swanson LM, Flynn H, Adams-Mundy JD, et al. An open pilot of cognitive-behavioral therapy for insomnia in women with postpartum depression. Behav Sleep Med 2013;11(4):297–307.
68. Sachs HC. The transfer of drugs and therapeutics into human breast milk: an update on selected topics. Pediatrics 2013;132(3):e796–809.

Management of Attention Deficit Hyperactivity Disorder During Pregnancy

Allison S. Baker, MD[a],*, Marlene P. Freeman, MD[b]

KEYWORDS

- Attention deficit hyperactivity disorder • Pregnancy • Methylphenidate
- Amphetamines

KEY POINTS

- Attention deficit hyperactivity disorder (ADHD) is one of the most common neurobehavioral disorders of childhood and commonly persists into adulthood.
- Women are increasingly using prescribed stimulant medications during pregnancy.
- ADHD symptoms affect daily functioning, including that of pregnant women with ADHD.
- Functional impairment can vary, and when moderate to severe, the benefit of stimulant medication use can outweigh risks of medication exposure (both known and unknown).
- If a decision is made to take ADHD medication, women should be informed of the known risks and benefits of the medication use in pregnancy, and take the lowest therapeutic dose possible; nonpharmacologic approaches should be maximized.

INTRODUCTION

Attention deficit hyperactivity disorder (ADHD) is one of the most common neurodevelopmental disorders of childhood, affecting about 3% to 7% of young people

Disclosure Statement: Dr A.S. Baker (current): Gerstner Family Foundation. Dr M.P. Freeman (current): investigator initiated trials (research): JayMac; research: Sage; Independent Data Safety and Monitoring Committee: Janssen (Johnson& Johnson); medical editing: GOED newsletter. Dr M.P. Freeman is an employee of Massachusetts General Hospital, and works with the MGH National Pregnancy Registry [current registry sponsors: Alkermes, Inc (2016-present); Otsuka America Pharmaceutical, Inc (2008-present); Forest/Actavis (2016-Present), Sunovion Pharmaceuticals, Inc (2011-Present)]. As an employee of MGH, Dr M.P. Freeman works with the MGH CTNI, which has had research funding from multiple pharmaceutical companies and National Institute of Mental Health.

a Perinatal and Reproductive Psychiatry Program, Harvard Medical School, Massachusetts General Hospital, 185 Cambridge Street, 2nd Floor, Boston, MA 02114, USA; b Perinatal and Reproductive Psychiatry Program, Harvard Medical School, CTNI, Women's Mental Health, Massachusetts General Hospital, 185 Cambridge Street, 2nd Floor, Boston, MA 02114, USA
* Corresponding author.
E-mail address: asbaker@mgh.harvard.edu

Obstet Gynecol Clin N Am 45 (2018) 495–509
https://doi.org/10.1016/j.ogc.2018.04.010
0889-8545/18/© 2018 Elsevier Inc. All rights reserved.

obgyn.theclinics.com

worldwide.[1] It is usually first diagnosed in childhood and often persists into adulthood,[2] with an estimated prevalence of ADHD in adult women of 3.2%.[3] Some individuals may have onset of the disorder during childhood, yet diagnosis and treatment might be delayed until later in life. This is of particular public health significance, because ADHD that persists into adulthood for women has been shown to be associated with depression, anxiety, self-injury, substance use, and occupational, social, and overall impairment domains.[4] Adult women with ADHD can experience a variety of difficulties at work and in their personal and family lives related to their ADHD symptoms.[5] Many experience relationship problems and may have chronic feelings of frustration, guilt, or blame.[6]

As a result, it is not surprising that ADHD is a diagnosis of concern and relevance in the pregnant population. As women plan for pregnancy, they seek to optimize their physical and mental health to yield the best outcomes possible from a maternal, fetal, and infant perspective. The US Centers for Disease Control and Prevention (CDC) have the following recommendations for women of reproductive age[7]:

- Take folic acid
- Maintain healthy diet and weight
- Regular physical activity
- Quit/abstain from tobacco use, alcohol, and drugs
- Communicate with health care providers about screening and management of chronic diseases
- Use effective contraception correctly if sexually active and wishing to delay/avoid pregnancy

It is important for obstetricians and gynecologists to familiarize themselves with the management of ADHD during pregnancy. Obstetricians and gynecologists benefit from an overview of the management of ADHD during pregnancy, because an increasing proportion of their patients present to obstetric care on ADHD medications.[8,9] Girls are being diagnosed and treated for ADHD at an earlier age, enhancing their opportunity to pursue higher education and achieve professional success. The gold standard treatment of ADHD is a combination of behavioral therapy and psychostimulant use, most often methylphenidate or amphetamine derivatives.[10] Many women continue their medication into their reproductive years, and need it for optimal functioning in the workplace setting or at home.

In addition to an understanding of the general risks and benefits of ADHD medications in pregnancy, specific attention is warranted to the relationship between the untreated disorder and substance abuse. In the field of obstetrics and gynecology, there are clear guidelines and recommendations about the importance of smoking cessation during pregnancy.[11] Importantly, untreated ADHD increases the risk for tobacco dependence.[12] Likewise, stimulant treatment for ADHD reduces the liability to addictive behaviors including maternal substance use disorders and tobacco dependence.[13]

To date, there have been no systematic reviews evaluating the course of ADHD across pregnancy and the postpartum period. There have been several systematic studies investigating perinatal exposure to stimulants,[14–16] although many of them are derived from data about women misusing ADHD medication, having multiple perinatal medication exposures, or medical comorbidities (including smoking).[17] This article will discuss management of ADHD during pregnancy including known and unknown risks of perinatal exposure to ADHD medication, and medical and psychiatric comorbidities.

PERINATAL PSYCHIATRIC CONSIDERATIONS

Although the default medical position is to interrupt any nonessential pharmacologic treatment during pregnancy and lactation, in ADHD this may present a significant risk. In the perinatal psychiatric consultation, the psychiatrist evaluates each case carefully and performs a risk-risk analysis with the patient prior to developing a treatment plan for pregnancy: the risks of medication exposure throughout the pregnancy weighed against the risks of untreated ADHD, including driving safety, and major impairment in fulfilling occupational and domestic roles.[18] To do this seamlessly, one would need a comprehensive reproductive safety literature that adequately controls for confounding variables. Unfortunately, this is far from the reality, especially in this clinical population. As such, studies often yield inconsistent results.[19] For example, some studies report concern for higher rates of miscarriage, low birth weight, shorter gestational ages, and low Apgar scores with prenatal methamphetamine exposure,[20–24] while other studies looking at the same prenatal medication exposure (methylphenidate) report no significant differences in rates of congenital malformations, median gestation age at delivery, rate of preterm delivery, or median birth weight.[25] Moreover, it is often the case that the same adverse outcome has been attributed to both a maternal mental disorder and a psychiatric medication.[25] The authors seek to clarify the evidence to date in **Fig. 1**, which summarizes inconsistent and real-world data of perinatal psychostimulant exposure across pregnancy. In particular, they highlight some areas of concern for an obstetrician seeing a pregnant woman with ADHD in the consultation room.

OBSTETRIC CONCERNS

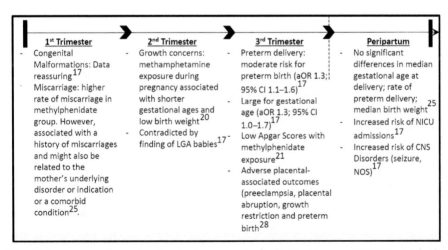

Fig. 1. Summary of psychostimulant exposure findings across pregnancy and the postpartum.

Case: A 32-Year-Old Attorney with Attention Deficit Hyperactivity Disorder Planning Pregnancy

Ms. C is a 32-year-old married attorney who presents for consultation regarding pregnancy planning. She has a diagnosis of ADHD combined type, first identified in first grade (age 6). She has been tried on a variety of stimulants, nonstimulants (atomoxetine, bupropion), and alpha-agonists (guanfacine) over the years. She reports the best she ever did was on methylphenidate extended release 40 mg daily. She has had trials off her medication between high school and college (gap year), college and law school (was clerking at a law firm), and between law school and her first job. All 3 trials off methylphenidate were characterized by significant difficulty functioning in her role (being late, misplacing items, forgetting appointments, and lack of attention to details warranting in a warning for poor work performance). As such, she notes that she is "very ambivalent" at the notion of stopping her medication, as she is the primary breadwinner for her family (husband is a teacher and is planning to be a stay at home dad when the baby is born).

Ms. C has done an extensive literature search on methylphenidate at the time of consultation. She is particularly concerned about risks to the baby being small for gestational age and hypertension. She asks if she could lower her dose and take weekends off her stimulant during pregnancy. She would like to breastfeed and will be granted a 16-week paid maternity leave with her current firm, during which time she would like to remain off methylphenidate.

After a consultation with Ms. C, her husband, and the psychiatrist, the decision is made to remain on her methylphenidate while attempting to conceive. Once she confirms a positive home pregnancy test, she plans to reduce her dose to methylphenidate immediate release 10 mg and use as necessary Monday through Thursday, and to take 1 work day (Fridays) and weekends off her stimulant medication during her pregnancy.

Ms. C conceived within 2 months of trying. She gained weight well during her pregnancy (25 pounds) and had healthy obstetric milestones, including a normal fetal anatomy scan, remaining normotensive, and demonstrating healthy growth of baby in utero. Ms. C began her maternity leave at 36 weeks' gestation and stopped her methylphenidate use at that time. Baby was born via normal spontaneous vaginal delivery (NSVD) at 40 weeks 2 days without complication (**Table 1**).

Risk-risk assessment

Ms. C and her psychiatrist performed a risk-risk assessment during the consultation to derive their clinical plan: weighing the risks of exposure to methylphenidate during pregnancy against the risks of Ms. C's ADHD symptoms roughening off stimulant medication. Ms. C and her husband briefly considered discontinuing her stimulant. However, Ms. C knew from experience that off methylphenidate altogether, there was a substantial risk of functional impairment in her role as an attorney, which was a professional and financial risk she was not able to tolerate. Furthermore, while Ms. C conceived rather quickly, another risk consideration in the risk-risk analysis was the possibility of it taking up to a year to conceive, and Ms. C felt that would not be feasible to remain off stimulants for that period of time due to the demanding nature of her profession.

Ms. C felt that by lowering her dose and using it more sparingly during the first trimester, she could mitigate risks of any potential cardiac malformations on methylphenidate.[26] She and her psychiatrist did wonder about switching to amphetamine (Adderall) based on the Huybrechts and colleagues (2017) study, but agreed that this was a risk in and of itself, as she had never tried Adderall and did not want to venture on a new medication trial during early pregnancy (that would invite risk of multiple medication exposures and risk of roughening of ADHD symptoms should amphetamine derivatives be ineffective for her). Ms. C, her psychiatrist, and her OB monitored her vital signs including blood pressure, and performed an ultrasound to ensure optimal fetal growth (minimizing risk of hypertensive disorders of pregnancy by close monitoring/ensuring healthy fetal growth).

Table 1
Studies investigating psychostimulant exposure during pregnancy

Author	Study Type	Exposed (n)	Psychostimulant	Summary	Confounding Variables[a]
Dideriksen et al,[15] 2013	Review	180	Methylphenidate (first trimester)	No indication for overall increased risk of congenital malformations ([RR] = 0.6; 95% CI, 0.2–1.6).	Accounted for (in regression model): alcohol, cigarette, and drug abuse and concurrent diseases
Källén et al,[22] 2013	Prospective, observational	208	Methylphenidate (early exposure)	Increased risk relative risk for cardiovascular malformations (relative risk [RR] = 1.81; 95% CI, 0.59–4.21)	Not accounted for: psychostimulant abuse
Haervig et al,[23] 2014	Population-based, cohort	480	Methylphenidate (81.88%), atomoxetime (9.38%), modafinil (8.75%)	Compared to the unexposed group, subjects using psychostimulant medication during pregnancy were demonstrated to have higher rates of elective termination as per maternal request (odds ratio = 4.70, 95% CI, 3.77–5.85), induced termination due to a special indication (odds ratio = 2.99; 95% CI, 1.34–6.67), and miscarriage (odds ratio = 2.07, 95% CI, 1.51–2.84).	Accounted for: age, ethnicity, region, psychostimulants specifically used for ADHD diagnosis. Additionally used a case-crossover analysis, which provided a comparison between exposed pregnancies to unexposed pregnancies of the same woman
Pottegård et al,[14] 2014	Population-based, cohort	222	Methylphenidate (first trimester)	No indication for overall increased risk of major malformations (point prevalence ratio = 0.8, 95% CI, 0.3–1.8) or cardiac malformations (point prevalence ratio = 0.9; 95% CI, 0.2–3.0).	Accounted for: use of drugs with documented teratogenicity, stimulants other than methylphenidate in exposed group

(continued on next page)

Table 1
(continued)

Author	Study Type	Exposed (n)	Psychostimulant	Summary	Confounding Variables[a]
Bro et al,[21] 2015	Population-based, cohort	186	Methylphenidate, atomoxetine	Compared with the unexposed group without an ADHD diagnosis, subjects using psychostimulant medication were demonstrated to have a higher risk of spontaneous termination (adjusted relative risk [aRR] = 1.55; 95% CI, 1.03–2.36). Infants born to mothers in this group also had an increased rate of <10 Apgar scores ([aRR] = 2.06; 95% CI, 1.11–3.82). Compared with the unexposed group without an ADHD diagnosis, women with ADHD who were unexposed to psychostimulant medication were also demonstrated to have a higher risk of spontaneous termination ([aRR] = 1.56; 95% CI, 1.11–2.20). Infants born to mothers in this group did not have an increased rate of <10 Apgar scores ([aRR] = 0.99; 95% CI, 0.48–2.05).	Accounted for: smoking, age, parity, use of other psychiatric drugs (ie, antipsychotic, antiepileptic, antidepressants), severity of mental disorder, drug misuse, epilepsy, comorbid depression

Diav-Citrin et al,[25] 2016	Prospective, comparative, multicenter observational	382	Methylphenidate (89.5% in first trimester)	No indication for overall increased risk of major malformations (6/247 = 2.4% exposed vs 12/358 = 3.4% unexposed, $P = .511$) or cardiac malformations (2/247 = 0.8% exposed vs 3/358 = 0.8 unexposed, $P = .970$) Compared with the unexposed group, subjects using methylphenidate demonstrated higher rates of miscarriage and elective terminations, with significant predictors including methylphenidate usage (adjusted hazard ratio [HR] = 1.98; 95% CI, 1.23–3.20; $P = .005$) and a previous miscarriage (adjusted [HR] = 1.35; 95% CI, 1.18–1.55; $P < .001$).	Accounted for: Gestational age at initial contact, maternal age, history of miscarriage, smoking, concomitant medications (ie, psychotropic drugs, nonsteroidal anti-inflammatory drugs)

(continued on next page)

Table 1
(continued)

Author	Study Type	Exposed (n)	Psychostimulant	Summary	Confounding Variables[a]
Newport et al,[24] 2016	Prospective, longitudinal observational study	12	2 Methylphenidate (n = 2), lisdexamphetamine (n = 1), amphetamine (n = 9) Post 20-wk gestation exposure	Hypertensive disorder of pregnancy associated with amphetamine exposure. Among the 9 women with post-PW20 amphetamine exposure, those diagnosed with HDP had significantly higher mean daily amphetamine doses (33.8 mg/d [95% CI, 17.6–50.1] vs 11.9 mg/d [95% CI, –2.2–25.9], t = 2.86, P = .02) and higher peak daily amphetamine doses (36.0 mg/d [95% CI, 17.2–54.8] vs 16.3 mg/d [95% CI, 4.3–28.2], t = 2.36, P = .05) after PW20 than those without HDP diagnoses. In patients in whom no alternatives are available, more vigilant prenatal monitoring for gestational hypertension is warranted.	Accounted for: Preexisting chronic hypertension, maternal age, ethnicity, obesity

| Nörby et al,[17] 2017 | Prospective, longitudinal | 1591 (0.2%) of 964734 infants in sample were exposed to ADHD medication during pregnancy (9475 infants (1.0%) had mothers treated before or after pregnancy) | Methylphenidate (~90% of exposed) | Exposure during pregnancy increased the risk for admission to a neonatal intensive care unit (NICU) compared with both no use and use before or after pregnancy (adjusted odds ratio [aOR], 1.5; 95% CI, 1.3–1.7; and aOR, 1.2; 95% CI, 1.1–1.4, respectively). Infants exposed during pregnancy had more often central nervous system–related disorders (aOR, 1.9; 95% CI, 1.1–3.1) and were more often moderately preterm (aOR, 1.3; 95% CI, 1.1–1.6) than nonexposed infants. There was no increased risk for congenital malformations or perinatal death. | Accounted for: birth year, maternal age, primiparity, BMI, maternal smoking, noncohabiting with father, mother born outside the Nordic countries, and use of opioids, antiepileptics, psycholeptics, antidepressants, alimemazine, or promethazine during pregnancy |

(continued on next page)

Table 1
(continued)

Author	Study Type	Exposed (n)	Psychostimulant	Summary	Confounding Variables[a]
Cohen et al,[29] 2017	Population-based, cohort	4846 stimulant exposure; 5299 including atomoxetine exposure	Amphetamine–dextroamphetamine (n = 3331), methylphenidate (n = 1515), and atomoxetine (a nonstimulant ADHD medication; n = 453) monotherapy in early pregnancy	Compared with the unexposed group, the exposed group had slightly increased risk of preeclampsia [aRR, 1.29; 95% CI, 1.11–1.49], placental abruption [aRR 1.13; 0.88–1.44], small gestational age [aRR 0.91; 0.77–1.07], and preterm birth [aRR 1.06; 0.97–1.16]. Psychostimulant continuation in the second half of pregnancy the risks were the following: preeclampsia [aRR, 1.26; 0.94–1.67], placental abruption [aRR 1.08; 0.67–1.74], small gestational age [aRR 1.37; 0.97–1.93], and preterm birth [aRR 1.30; 1.10–1.55]. These findings were not associated with atomoxetine usage.	Accounted for: age, race, geographic region, year at assessment, multiparity, multifetal gestation, alcohol use or drug use/abuse/dependency, obesity, chronic health conditions (inflammatory, cardiovascular, renal), stimulant indication and indication severity, additional psychiatric and pain conditions, proxies for health care utilization intensity, and cotreatment with psychiatric and pain medication

| Huybrechts et al,[26] 2017 | Population-based, cohort | 7643 | Methylphenidate (n = 2072) and amphetamine (n = 5571) exposures during the first 90 d of pregnancy | Cardiac malformations risk per 1000 infants: Nonexposed:12.7 (95%CI, 12.6–12.9) Methylphenidate: 18.8 (95%CI, 13.8–25.6) Amphetamines: 15.4 (95% CI, 12.5–19.0) Adjusted relative risks for methylphenidate: 1.11 (95% CI, 0.91–1.35) for any malformation and 1.28 (95% CI, 0.94–1.74) for cardiac malformations. No increased risks were observed for amphetamines: 1.05 (95% CI, 0.93–1.19) for any malformations and 0.96 (95% CI, 0.78–1.19) for cardiac malformations. Replication analysis for methylphenidate using the Nordic data (n = 2,560,069) pregnancies yielded a relative risk of 1.28 (95% CI, 0.83–1.97) for cardiac malformations, resulting in a pooled estimate of 1.28 (95% CI, 1.00–1.64). | Accounted for: Excluded pregnancies exposed to known teratogens and with chromosomal abnormalities Age, race/ethnicity, year of delivery, multiparity, multiple gestations, psychiatric conditions, chronic comorbid medical conditions, markers of general comorbidity, prescribed medications (including other psychotropic medications, antidiabetic and antihypertensive medications, suspected teratogens, as well as proxies for drug abuse or dependence) |

a Some covariates included in analysis may not have been explicitly stated in the text and instead were included in supplemental materials and/or databases.

MANAGEMENT GOALS

In order to optimize maternal functioning and minimize risk in terms of unnecessary exposure to fetus, goals should include

- Prevent roughening of comorbid mood and anxiety disorders
- Coordination of care between providers: obstetrics/gynecology and psychiatry
- Routine vital signs checks including blood pressure and assessment of adequate weight gain

PHARMACOLOGIC STRATEGIES

Stimulants options include

- Methylphenidate
- Amphetamine
- Dexamphetamine
- Lisdexamfetamine

Nonstimulant medication options include bupropion and atomoxetine.

In some cases, prenatally switching from stimulant medication to bupropion may be a middle path to walk in terms of targeting ADHD symptoms and comorbid depression. Prospective birth outcome data that are available in the Bupropion Pregnancy Registry suggest that birth defect rates with bupropion exposure are similar to that of the general population,[27] although it is not as efficacious as stimulants in the treatment of ADHD.[28]

In a 2017 population-based cohort study, women receiving atomoxetine (453) were not at risk for preeclampsia, placental abruption, small for gestation age status, or preterm birth.[29]

BREASTFEEDING

There are limited data available to inform patients and practitioners about the use of psychostimulants during breastfeeding. In dosages prescribed for medical indications (as opposed to stimulants of abuse), some evidence indicates that dextroamphetamine might not affect nursing infants adversely.[30] In 2 infants, the plasma level of dextroamphetamine was low but detectable, while in the third it was undetectable.

Table 2 Adjustment and recurrence strategy for attention deficit hyperactivity disorder during pregnancy		
Mild ADHD (Minimal Functional Impairment off Medication)	Moderate ADHD (Some Functional Impairment off Medication)	Severe ADHD (Significant Functional Impairment, Including Driving Safety)
Optimize sufficient nonpharmacologic management strategies and ensure self-management strategies in place (with history of success in supporting functionality of woman in domestic and occupational roles)	Optimize nonpharmacologic strategies; consider when necessary use of stimulant	Maintain medication, consider closer obstetric monitoring for fetal growth and hypertensive disorders of pregnancy

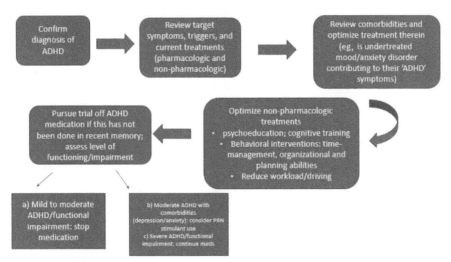

Fig. 2. Explanatory algorithm for clinicians working with pregnant patients with ADHD.

The mean infant dose assessed was 5.7% of the maternal dose, below the 10% cutoff usually cited in the breastfeeding literature as relatively low. The estimated infant dose was lower (0.16%–0.2%) in 2 other case reports of infants who were breastfed while the mothers were treated with methylphenidate.[31]

NONPHARMACOLOGIC STRATEGIES

There have been studies of psychotherapeutic approaches for ADHD. Cognitive behavioral therapy (CBT) has been demonstrated to have a significant impact on symptoms.[32]

CBT and coaching strategies can help improve functioning, and assist the individual in tailoring routines in ways to cope with ADHD. For some women, these strategies may be enough to improve functioning without the need for medication.

Self-management strategies include reducing the workload if possible and taking public transportation instead of driving. Options must be evaluated regularly and adjusted if needed, especially if symptoms recur. Physicians should have a strategy in mind should symptoms recur (**Table 2**). **Fig. 2** has an explanatory algorithm for clinicians working with pregnant patients with ADHD.

SUMMARY

ADHD is a common neurobehavioral disorder of childhood and adulthood. It is associated with significant psychiatric comorbidities for women, including depression, anxiety, substance use disorders, driving safety impairment, and occupational impairment. The gold standard treatment includes behavioral therapy and stimulant medication, namely methylphenidate and amphetamine derivatives. Psychostimulant use during pregnancy continues to increase and has been associated with a small increased relative risk of a range of obstetric concerns. However, the absolute increases in risks are small, and many of the best studies to date are confounded by other medication use and medical comorbidities. Thus, women with moderate-to-severe ADHD should not necessarily be counseled to suspend their ADHD treatment based on these findings. Of note, long-term neurobehavioral data on prenatal exposure to psychostimulants remain lacking, so management during pregnancy must be weighed against that unknown risk.

ACKNOWLEDGMENTS

The authors would like to thank Olivia Noe for her invaluable editorial assistance in the preparation of this article.

REFERENCES

1. Thomas R, Sanders S, Doust J, et al. Prevalence of attention-deficit/hyperactivity disorder: a systematic review and meta-analysis. Pediatrics 2015;135(4): e994–1001.
2. Cho SW, Lee YJ, Lee SA, et al. Comparison of adults with attention-deficit hyperactivity disorder depending on the age of being diagnosed in childhood and adulthood: based on retrospective review in one university hospital. Journal of the Korean Academy of Child and Adolescent Psychiatry 2017;28(3):183–9.
3. Kessler RC, Adler L, Barkley R, et al. The prevalence and correlates of adult ADHD in the United States: results from the National Comorbidity Survey Replication. Am J Psychiatry 2006;163(4):716–23.
4. Owens EB, Zalecki C, Gillette P, et al. Girls with childhood ADHD as adults: cross-domain outcomes by diagnostic persistence. J Consult Clin Psychol 2017. https://doi.org/10.1037/ccp0000217.
5. Corbisiero S, Hartmann-Schorro RM, Riecher-Rössler A, et al. Screening for adult attention-deficit/hyperactivity disorder in a psychiatric outpatient population with specific focus on sex differences. Front Psychiatry 2017;8:115.
6. Eddy LD, Jones HA, Snipes D, et al. Associations between ADHD symptoms and occupational, interpersonal, and daily life impairments among pregnant women. J Atten Disord 2017. https://doi.org/10.1177/1087054716685839. 1087054716685839.
7. Centers for Disease Control and Prevention. Unintended pregnancy prevention: home. Washington DC: United States Department of Health and Human Services; 2010. Available at: http://www.cdc.gov/reproductivehealth/UnintendedPregnancy/index.htm.
8. Leong C, Raymond C, Château D, et al. Psychotropic drug use before, during, and after pregnancy: a population-based study in a Canadian cohort (2001-2013). Can J Psychiatry 2017. https://doi.org/10.1177/0706743717711168. 0706743717711168.
9. Louik C, Kerr S, Kelley KE, et al. Increasing use of ADHD medications in pregnancy. Pharmacoepidemiol Drug Saf 2015;24(2):218.
10. Thapar A, Cooper M. Attention deficit hyperactivity disorder. Lancet 2018; 387(10024):1240–50.
11. Committee on Obstetric Practice. Committee Opinion No. 721: Smoking cessation during pregnancy. Obstetrics and Gynecology 2017;130(4):e200.
12. Kollins SH, McClernon FJ, Fuemmeler BF. Association between smoking and attention-deficit/hyperactivity disorder symptoms in a population-based sample of young adults. Arch Gen Psychiatry 2005;62(10):1142–7.
13. Groenman AP, Oosterlaan J, Rommelse NN, et al. Stimulant treatment for attention-deficit hyperactivity disorder and risk of developing substance use disorder. Br J Psychiatry 2013;203(2):112–9.
14. Pottegård A, Hallas J, Andersen JT, et al. First-trimester exposure to methylphenidate: a population-based cohort study. J Clin Psychiatry 2014;75(1):e88–93.

15. Dideriksen D, Pottegård A, Hallas J, et al. First trimester in utero exposure to methylphenidate. Basic Clin Pharmacol Toxicol 2013;112(2):73–6.
16. Wajnberg R, Diav-Citrin O, Shechtman S, et al. Pregnancy outcome after in-utero exposure to methylphenidate: a prospective comparative cohort study. Reprod Toxicol 2011;31(2):267.
17. Nörby U, Winbladh B, Källén K. Perinatal outcomes after treatment with ADHD medication during pregnancy. Pediatrics 2017;e20170747. https://doi.org/10. 1542/peds.2017-0747.
18. Freeman MP. ADHD and pregnancy. Am J Psychiatry 2014;171(7):723–8.
19. Newport DJ, Fernandez SV, Juric S, et al. Psychopharmacology during pregnancy and lactation. In: Schatzberg AF, Nemeroff CB, editors. The American psychiatric publishing textbook of psychopharmacology. 4th Edition. Washington, DC: American Psychiatric Publishing, Inc; 2009. p. 1373.
20. Wright TE, Schuetter R, Tellei J, et al. Methamphetamines and pregnancy outcomes. J Addict Med 2015;9(2):111.
21. Bro SP, Kjaersgaard MI, Parner ET, et al. Adverse pregnancy outcomes after exposure to methylphenidate or atomoxetine during pregnancy. Clin Epidemiol 2015;7:139.
22. Källén B, Borg N, Reis M. The use of central nervous system active drugs during pregnancy. Pharmaceuticals (Basel) 2013;6(10):1221–86.
23. Haervig KB, Mortensen LH, Hansen AV, et al. Use of ADHD medication during pregnancy from 1999 to 2010: a Danish register-based study. Pharmacoepidemiol Drug Saf 2014;23(5):526–33.
24. Newport DJ, Hostetter AL, Juul SH, et al. Prenatal psychostimulant and antidepressant exposure and risk of hypertensive disorders of pregnancy. J Clin Psychiatry 2016;77(11):1538–45.
25. Diav-Citrin O, Shechtman S, Arnon J, et al. Methylphenidate in pregnancy: a multicenter, prospective, comparative, observational study. J Clin Psychiatry 2016;77(9):1176–81.
26. Huybrechts KF, Bröms G, Christensen LB, et al. Association between methylphenidate and amphetamine use in pregnancy and risk of congenital malformations: a cohort study from the International Pregnancy Safety Study Consortium. JAMA Psychiatry 2017. https://doi.org/10.1001/jamapsychiatry.2017.3644.
27. GlaxoSmithKline. The Bupropion Pregnancy Registry. Final report. 1 September 1997 through 31 March 2008. Wilmington (NC): Kendle International Inc; 2008.
28. Peterson K, McDonagh MS, Fu R. Comparative benefits and harms of competing medications for adults with attention-deficit hyperactivity disorder: a systematic review and indirect comparison meta-analysis. Psychopharmacology (Berl) 2008;197(1):1–11.
29. Cohen JM, Hernández-Díaz S, Bateman BT, et al. Placental complications associated with psychostimulant use in pregnancy. Obstet Gynecol 2017. https://doi. org/10.1097/AOG.0000000000002362.
30. Ilett KF, Hackett LP, Kristensen JH, et al. Transfer of dexamphetamine into breast milk during treatment for attention deficit hyperactivity disorder. Br J Clin Pharmacol 2007;63(3):371–5.
31. Spigset O, Brede WR, Zahlsen K. Excretion of methylphenidate in breast milk. Am J Psychiatry 2007;164(2):348.
32. Mongia M, Hechtman L. Cognitive behavior therapy for adults with attention-deficit/hyperactivity disorder: a review of recent randomized controlled trials. Curr Psychiatry Rep 2012;14(5):561–7.

Treatment of Perinatal Opioid Use Disorder

Lisa Boyars, MD[a], Constance Guille, MD, MSCR[a,b,*]

KEYWORDS

- Opioid use disorder • Pregnancy • Medication-assisted withdrawal • Buprenorphine
- Methadone • Opioid agonist therapy

KEY POINTS

- Identification of perinatal opioid use disorder is improved by using validated screening questionnaires, understanding the limitations of urine drug screens, reviewing prescription drug monitoring programs, and nonjudgmental clinical care.
- Opioid agonist therapy is the standard of care for pregnant women with Opioid Use Disorder, however medication- assisted withdrawal is an increasingly common practice.
- Based on available data and addiction clinical care, we provide guidance for obstetricians to assist pregnant women in making an informed medication treatment choice that is best for women and their families.
- Choosing a treatment to assist pregnant women in their recovery ultimately produces the best outcome for women and their children.

INTRODUCTION

The epidemic of opioid use, misuse, and opioid use disorder (OUD) in the United States is well-known to extend into pregnancy. Prescription opioids are dispensed by pharmacies to 14.4% to 21.1% of all pregnant women.[1,2] Pregnant women dispensed 2 or more prescription opioids suggesting a long-term pattern of opioid use, occurs in 3% to 5% of women and has increased 4-fold over the past decade.[1] The prevalence of opioid abuse or dependence among pregnant women has more than doubled from 1.7 per 1000 deliveries in 1998 to 3.9 per 1000 deliveries in 2011 with the most substantial increase occurring in 20- to 34-year-old women.[3] All indications are that these rates are still rising.

Disclosure Statement: The authors report no direct financial interest in subject matter or materials discussed in article or with a company making a competing product.
[a] Department of Psychiatry and Behavioral Sciences, Medical University of South Carolina, MSC 861, 67 President Street, Charleston, SC 29403, USA; [b] Department of Obstetrics and Gynecology, Medical University of South Carolina, MSC 861, 67 President Street, Charleston, SC 29403, USA
* Corresponding author. Department of Psychiatry and Behavioral Sciences, MSC 861, 67 President Street, Charleston SC 29403.
E-mail address: guille@musc.edu

Perinatal OUD is a major public health problem because of its impact on maternal, fetal, newborn, and child health, as well as excessive use of health care resources.[3,4] Extant literature describing the maternal, obstetric, and newborn risks associated with OUD is well-established and is associated with a 4.6-fold increased risk for maternal death at delivery as well as an increased risk for intrauterine growth restriction, placental abruption, prematurity, blood transfusion, stillbirth, cesarean delivery, pre-eclampsia, or eclampsia.[3] A well-known consequence of opioid use in pregnancy is newborn opioid withdrawal syndrome (NOWS), formally known as neonatal absti-nence syndrome, with 60% of newborns exhibiting withdrawal symptoms after deliv-ery.[4] Over the past decade, the incidence of NOWS in the United States has increased approximately 400%, from 1.2 per 1000 hospital births in 2000 to 5.8 per 1000 hospital births in 2012. In 2012, on average, 1 infant was born every 25 minutes in the United States with signs of opioid withdrawal, costing $1.5 billion dollars, with Medicaid covering 80% of these costs.[4]

Despite the significant and costly maternal, fetal, and newborn effects of perinatal OUD, there is a paucity of comprehensive treatment programs for pregnant women with substance use disorders.[5–7] Only 19 states have funded substance abuse treat-ment programs for pregnant women, and only 12 states provide priority to pregnant women to receive substance abuse treatment.[5–7] Further, stigma is a potent barrier to care as well as lack of adequate childcare and fear of criminal or child welfare con-sequences.[5] As a result, few pregnant women receive treatment for substance use disorders during pregnancy.

The challenges of identifying, managing, and treating OUD combined with the paucity of treatment resources for this population places an unfair burden on front-line obstetricians. Additionally, treatment with opioid agonist therapy (eg, methadone or buprenorphine) versus medication-assisted withdrawal is controversial. Front-line providers are currently providing care to this population and would greatly benefit from practical clinical guidance based on the current evidence.

In this article, we provide front-line providers with practical clinical information to assist in the identification and treatment of pregnant women with OUD. In addition, we review the evidence to date examining the risks and benefits of opioid agonist ther-apy and medication-assisted withdrawal for the treatment of perinatal OUD. We pro-vide practical clinical tools for patients and providers to help guide medication treatment choices. We provide further guidance on how to counsel patients about these treatment choices as well as the need for relapse prevention therapy and regular follow-up care for the treatment of OUD.

SCREENING FOR SUBSTANCE USE
Validated Screening Questionnaires

Early identification of pregnant women with opioid use is vital to improving outcomes for mothers, infants, and children. National and international organizations including the American College of Obstetricians and Gynecologists, Substance Abuse and Mental Health Services Administration, American Society for Addiction Medicine, World Health Organization, and United Nations recommend routine universal screening for substance use performed in partnership, and with the consent of, preg-nant women using brief validated screening tools and mutual dialogue.[8–14] These pro-fessional organizations recommend screening at the initial prenatal care visit, and at several points throughout prenatal care, to facilitate the early identification and imple-mentation of comprehensive prenatal and substance abuse treatment.[8,10,11,15] Although there are many validated instruments to screen for alcohol use during pregnancy, there are few validated instruments to screen for opiate use. The 4P's Plus, National Institute on Drug Abuse Quick Screen, and CRAFFT are validated screening instruments in pregnant populations and are currently recommended for use by professional organizations (**Table 1**).[15]

Although it has not been validated in pregnant populations to date, Screening, Brief Intervention and Referral to Treatment is an evidence-based practice that is used to screen and identify problematic alcohol and illicit drug use and assist in brief intervention and appropriate referral to treatment. Reimbursement for SIBRT exists through private insurers and Medicaid; however, there are some limitations on number of Screening, Brief Intervention and Referral to Treatment-related visits that qualify. Screening, Brief Intervention and Referral to Treatment can be performed by clinical staff after minimal training under direction of a physician, or by the physicians themselves.

Prescription Drug Monitoring Program

The prescription drug monitoring program is a state electronic database that tracks controlled prescriptions filled by pharmacies and can be a helpful resource in identifying the use of controlled substances, such as prescription opioids, stimulants, or benzodiazepines. The wide availability of prescription drug monitoring programs can be a helpful tool in identifying patients filling prescriptions for controlled substances from multiple sources. It is helpful to review the prescription drug monitoring program in advance of meeting with the patient and using the clinical interview to clarify prescriptions that suggest a potential for prescription misuse or abuse, such as receiving early medication refills, having multiple providers, overlapping prescriptions, and/or escalating dosage of medication over time. It is also important to note methadone dispensed from a methadone treatment center is not registered in the prescription drug monitoring program.

Clinical Interview

Assessment of substance use using a clinical interview should take place after the completion of self-report assessments and review of the prescription drug monitoring program. The clinical interview should be conducted in a private office with a closed door and can include the aforementioned interview-based questionnaires. Phillips and colleagues[16] investigated factors that influence the disclosure of substance use during pregnancy. Investigators identified practice styles that include a nonjudgmental, supportive, caring, direct, and honest approach as the most helpful in facilitating the disclosure of perinatal substance use. Showing encouragement and praise also enhanced rapport and discussion of perinatal substance use.[16] It is important to be sensitive to the fact that women may fear that disclosure of substance use will result in losing custody of their child. Addressing this issue directly by informing women of any state mandatory requirements and any local procedures that will occur during pregnancy and/or at the time of delivery will help the patient and provider to plan for the best course of action, including the treatment of substance use disorders during pregnancy as opposed to waiting for this step to be identified and addressed at delivery or postpartum. It is critical to be aware of the local substance abuse and mental health treatment options in your area as well as acknowledge their limitations so that a plan for treatment can be made immediately.

The presence of at least 2 of the criteria are present over the past 12 months as described in the *Diagnostic and Statistical Manual of Mental Disorders, Fifth Edition*[17] that can be categorized by an inability to control one's use of a substance resulting in significant occupational and relational and/or social impairment, as well as other risk

Table 1
Substance use screening instruments for pregnant women

	4P's Plus[a]	NIDA Quick Screen	CRAFFT[b]
Number of questions	5	4	6
Patient population	Pregnant women	Pregnant women ≥18 y	Pregnant women ≤26 y
Questions	*Parents:* Did either of your parents ever have a problem with alcohol or drugs? *Partner:* Does your partner have a problem with alcohol or drugs? *Past:* Have you ever drunk beer, wine, or liquor? *Pregnancy:* In the month before you knew you were pregnant, how many cigarettes did you smoke? In the month before you knew you were pregnant, how many beers/how much wine/how much liquor did you drink?	In the past year how often have you used the following? 1. Alcohol (≥4 drinks in a day) 2. Tobacco products 3. Prescription drugs for nonmedical reasons 4. Illegal drugs Answer choice options include never, once or twice monthly, weekly, daily or almost daily	Part A: During the past 12 months, on how many days did you: 1. Drink more than a few sips of beer, wine, or any drink containing alcohol? 2. Use any marijuana (pot, weed, hash, or in foods) or "synthetic marijuana" (like "K2" or "Spice")? 3. Use anything else to get high (like other illegal drugs, prescription or over-the-counter medication, and things that you sniff or "huff")? If the patient answers "0" for all Part A questions, then ask CAR questions only. Otherwise, ask all 6 CRAFFT questions below. Part B: C: Have you ever ridden in a CAR driven by someone (including yourself) who was "high" or had been using alcohol or drugs? R: Do you ever use alcohol or drugs to RELAX, feel better about yourself, or fit in? A: Do you use alcohol or drugs while you are by yourself or ALONE? F: Do you ever FORGET things you did while using alcohol or drugs? F: Do your FAMILY or FRIENDS ever tell you that you should cut down on your drinking or drug use? T: Have you ever gotten in TROUBLE while you were using alcohol or drugs?
Positive screening	If positive, proceed to more structured clinical assessment for substance use	If positive, begin NIDA Modified ASSIST	If positive (score >2 or 3), proceed to more structured clinical assessment for substance use

Abbreviation: NIDA, National Institute on Drug Abuse.

of harm to one's self. Tolerance and withdrawal alone do not support the diagnosis of an OUD and are considered a normal physiologic effect of opioid use.

Urine Drug Screen

A urine drug screen (UDS) should only be completed after screening and a clinical interview, and is used to support the clinical diagnosis. A UDS cannot establish the presence of a substance use disorder. A clinical interview is used to make this diagnosis. Ideally, a validated screening instrument paired with a clinical interview and a UDS can be completed to support the diagnosis at the first prenatal visit and periodically thereafter.[15]

It is important for providers to recognize the limitation of the UDS in that most do not detect synthetic and semisynthetic opioids like oxycodone, hydrocodone, buprenorphine, and oxymorphone.[18–20] These drugs go unrecognized on standard urine enzyme-linked immunoassays (EIAs). Practitioners should be familiar with the toxicology laboratory screens that they use and test for specific semisynthetic opiates or their metabolites via EIA when appropriate.[21,22] Gas chromatography-mass spectrometry is the most accurate, sensitive, and reliable means of drug testing. It is generally performed after a positive result from immunoassay because it is time consuming and costly. Although gas chromatography-mass spectrometry is standard for confirmatory drug testing, it can fail to identify a positive specimen if the column is designed to detect only certain substances.

UDS are subject to cross-reactivity potentially causing a false-positive result with other opioid and nonopioid medications; unfortunately, the actual prevalence of false-positive results are unclear. Morphine, methadone, codeine, dihydrocodeine, and morphine-3-glucuronide may all produce positive results for buprenorphine EIAs.[23] Morphine is a metabolic byproduct of heroin, so it is possible to test positive for both heroin and morphine when using heroin. Additionally, some nonopioid medications, including diphenhydramine, several fluoroquinolones, quietapine, and verapamil, have been evaluated for cross-reactivity and tested positive on certain EIAs for methadone.[24] If you suspect cross-reactivity, gas chromatography-mass spectrometry should be ordered to determine the presence of absence of an opioid medication. Another limitation of the UDS is that the drugs and metabolites are only detectable in urine for a short duration. **Table 2** provides a reference and estimate for the amount of time opioids can be detected in urine for commonly used opioids.[25]

TREATMENT OF OPIOID USE DISORDER
Therapy

Treatment for OUD includes psychosocial interventions geared toward motivational enhancement and relapse prevention.[26] Through a combination of relapse prevention

Table 2	
Amount of time opioid can be detected in urine after ingestion	
Codeine	48 h
Heroin (morphine)	48 h
Hydromorphone	2–4 d
Methadone	3 d
Morphine	2–3 d
Oxycodone	2–4 d

Adapted from Moeller KE, Lee KC, Kissack JC. Urine drug screening: practical guide for clinicians. Mayo Clin Proc 2008;83(1):67; with permission.

therapy, 12-step programs, and increased family, social and community supports, patients are better able to keep recovery and primary motivators for change in the forefront of their treatment.[27] It is important to recognize that the vast majority of women with substance use have significant histories of trauma, and health care providers that are trained in trauma-informed care create a safe environment for these patients that enhance rapport and engagement in treatment.[28] (Please see Dr Florian's article, "The Unwelcome Guest: Working with Childhood Sexual Abuse Survivors in Reproductive Health Care," in this issue). Patient with significant trauma histories should be evaluated for posttraumatic stress disorder and referred for trauma-focused therapy with a qualified provider.

Opioid Agonist Therapy Versus Medication-Assisted Withdrawal

Before the prescription opioid epidemic, opioid agonist therapy with either methadone or buprenorphine, combined with drug counseling, was the standard of care for pregnant women with OUD.[9] This recommendation is based on data collected before 2002 and primarily included women with intravenous opioid and/or heroin use. Collectively, these data demonstrated that 41% to 96% of pregnant women relapsed to drug use, or convert to taking methadone if opioid agonist therapy is discontinued, with poor obstetric outcomes related to relapse to drug use.[29–33] One study that compared methadone with medication-assisted withdrawal demonstrated that those receiving methadone remained in treatment longer (110 vs 20 days), attended more obstetric care visits (8.3 vs 2.3), and were more likely to deliver at the hospital associated with their addiction treatment program.[32] Although there are obstetric and newborn risks associated with opioid agonist therapy such as prematurity, low birth weight, and newborn opioid withdrawal,[9] relapse to intravenous or illicit drug use places women at even greater risk for poor obstetric outcomes, as well as sexually transmitted infections, hepatitis, sepsis, and cellulitis, and may leave women susceptible to prostitution, theft, violence, and other legal consequences associated with illegal drug use.[34] Therefore, most experts conclude that the risks of relapse to drug use far outweigh the risks of opioid agonist medications.[9,35]

It is unknown, however, if opioid agonist therapy is superior to medication-assisted withdrawal for contemporary populations with OUD that primarily involves nonintravenous use of prescription opioids. The majority of those who abuse prescription opioids report using opioids orally, not intravenously, do not have a history of heroin use, and use smaller amounts of opioids per day, compared with those with heroin use.[36] Therefore, those with primarily prescription opioid use are less likely to have the aforementioned risks associated with intravenous and illicit drug use. Recent data suggest that buprenorphine can be discontinued in pregnancy with little obvious obstetric or fetal risk and potentially a reduced risk of newborn withdrawal.[37,38] In 1 study, infants born to mothers who underwent medication-assisted withdrawal had significantly lower NOWS peak scores, required less morphine to treat NOWS, had fewer days medicated for NOWS, and remained in the hospital for a shorter duration.[39] Another study found that the birth weight of neonates was significantly higher for women who had tapered their opiate maintenance treatment dose by more than 50% compared with women who did not taper their dose during pregnancy.[38]

However, it continues to be uncertain if pregnant women with prescription OUD who undergo medication-assisted withdrawal are at high risk for either relapse to prescription opioid use or other illicit drug use. Since 2002, there have been 5 studies including a total of 613 pregnant women with OUD who have attempted medication-assisted withdrawal.[37–41] Two national cohort studies completed in Norway[38] and

Canada[41] reviewed the maternal and newborn outcomes of opioid-dependent women participating in outpatient opioid maintenance programs, which decreased their medication dose during pregnancy. A range of 40% to 80% of pregnant women with OUD were able to reduce their maintenance opioid medication, and approximately 2% to 10% were able to completely stop opioid medication during pregnancy. At the time of delivery, 50% to 100% were successful at using only the reduced medication dosage and had favorable newborn outcomes.[38,41] In a small study comparing methadone (n = 12) and buprenorphine (n = 5) with methadone-assisted withdrawal (n = 8) during pregnancy, there were no differences between groups in obstetric outcomes or UDS positivity at the time of delivery.[40] In a retrospective cohort study of 95 pregnant women with opioid use, more than one-half of women were successful in detoxification after inpatient hospitalization. Women with longer durations of detoxification hospital stays and those who completed the entire detoxification program remained opioid free at delivery.[39] Bell and colleagues[37] reported no increased risk for poor obstetric outcomes among 301 pregnant women with OUD who discontinued buprenorphine during pregnancy, even with vastly different withdrawal protocols, including abrupt cessation with symptomatic treatment (n = 108 incarcerated women), a 5- to 10-day inpatient buprenorphine-assisted withdrawal protocol (n = 100 women), and a 6- to 12-week outpatient buprenorphine-assisted withdrawal protocol (n = 93 women). These groups differed, however, in risk for relapse, with the greatest risk for those with little to no outpatient care after inpatient detoxification (77%). Rates of relapse to opioid use was 17.2% among women who completed an inpatient taper followed by discharge to a group home, and 17.4% among women completing an outpatient taper with intensive outpatient follow-up care.

Taken together, these data suggest that women can decrease or discontinue their use of opioid agonist therapy during pregnancy with a low risk for poor obstetric and newborn outcomes. Plus, there is a low risk for relapse to drug use for those receiving longer and more intensive follow-up care. However, the characteristics of optimal care for pregnant women with prescription OUD who choose medication-assisted withdrawal are poorly defined and methodologic limitations of prior studies decrease our ability to draw definitive conclusions. Studies to date are retrospective, underpowered, and lack detailed maternal, placental, fetal, and newborn assessments or adequate control groups. Prospective, well-powered studies that systematically assess critical maternal, placental, fetal, and newborn outcomes among women who choose to discontinue their opioid agonist therapy compared with those who continue this therapy are greatly needed.

Given the current burden of neonatal opioid withdrawal syndrome, limited patient access to opioid agonist treatment, and usual patient preference to discontinue this therapy during pregnancy,[4–7] women frequently choose medication-assisted withdrawal without considering their potential risk for relapse to drug use and the associated consequences. Women would benefit from discussing with their front-line obstetricians what is currently known and unknown about the perinatal risks, as well as maternal risk of relapse with tapering opioid agonist therapy in general, and for the individual woman.

The clinical parameters described in **Table 3** can assist clinicians in these discussions and helping women to choose the best treatment option given the current literature and their addiction history. In particular, we describe the characteristics of those who are potentially good candidates for opioid agonist treatment or medication-assisted withdrawal. For each of these choices, we provide suggestions of issues that the patient and provider should consider.

Table 3
Opioid use disorder medication treatment options: patient eligibility, counseling, and education

Taper	Buprenorphine	Methadone
Eligibility		
• Inpatient or outpatient treatment • No history of IVDU • No access to opioid agonist therapy • Patient preference to not take opioid agonist therapy	• Office-based or inpatient buprenorphine induction • Available providers to prescribe buprenorphine • Amenable to and compliant with outpatient treatment	• Federally designated clinics • History of IVDU or severe opioid use disorder • Failed buprenorphine or unable to tolerate buprenorphine • Prior benefit from methadone
Counseling and patient–physician agreement		
• Patient–physician agreement • Aware of treatment options • Understands risk of relapse • Understands risks and benefits of medication-assisted withdrawal and opioid agonist therapy • Willing to engage in relapse prevention therapy • Positive social supports • Few psychosocial stressors • Plan for how to manage cravings or relapse • Encourage breastfeeding, as long as patient not using other illicit substances, or HIV positive	• Patient–physician agreement • Aware of treatment options • Understands risk of relapse • Understands the risks and benefits of buprenorphine • Willing to engage in relapse prevention therapy • Use caution with CNS depressants • Encourage breastfeeding, as long as patient not using other illicit substances, or HIV positive	• Patient–physician agreement • Aware of treatment options • Understands risk of relapse • Understands risk and benefits of methadone • Use caution with other agents that prolong the QTc interval • Encourage breastfeeding, as long as patient not using other illicit substances, or HIV positive
Prescription and monitoring		
• Ensure that patient is engaged in relapse prevention • Lower dose by no more than 20% of the initial starting dose per week[31] • Monitor cravings, stress, and other drug use • If reporting craving and/or drug use increase dose to prior effective dose, split daily dose, or try more gradual taper • Random UDS	• Ensure that patient is engaged in relapse prevention • Monitor cravings, stress, and other drug use • Increase dose if reporting cravings, physical withdrawal symptoms, or drug use • Random UDS	• Ensure that patient is engaged in relapse prevention • Monitor cravings, stress, and other drug use • Increase dose if reporting cravings, physical withdrawal symptoms, or drug use • Random UDS
Psychoeducation		
• Monitor abstinence via patient self-report and UDS • Manage withdrawal symptoms with either reducing the rate or dose of medication taper and/or use split daily dosing.	• Monitor abstinence via patients self-report and UDS • Lower risk of overdose than methadone • Few drug interactions	• Monitor abstinence via patient self-report and UDS • Get pretreatment QTc, follow-up in 30 d, and then annually

(continued on next page)

Table 3 (continued)		
Taper	**Buprenorphine**	**Methadone**
• Withdrawal symptoms can also be managed with symptomatic treatments: metoprolol for tachycardia, Phenergan for nausea, dicyclomine for loose stool, and cyclobenzaprine for muscle spasm • Recommend 12-step programs and relapse prevention	• Patient must be in withdrawal for buprenorphine induction • Risk for NOWS • Recommend 12 step programs and relapse prevention	• Risk for NOWS • Recommend 12-step programs and relapse prevention

Abbreviations: CNS, central nervous system; HIV, human immunodeficiency virus; IVDU, intravenous drug use; NOWS, newborn opioid withdrawal syndrome; UDS, urine drug screen.

Methadone and Buprenorphine

As mentioned, opioid agonist therapy is the standard of care for pregnant women with Opioid Use Disorder. This recommendation is well-supported by prior literature.[9,29–33,35] Methadone and buprenorphine are good treatment options with both having advantages for certain patients. Among nonpregnant populations, good candidates for treatment with methadone are those with severe addiction, or unsuccessful abstinence from drug use with buprenorphine or those who would benefit from the structure and support of daily observed therapy at a methadone treatment center.[27] Women who are able to adhere to outpatient therapy with less structure are typically good candidates for buprenorphine.[27] Buprenorphine may be a good first choice for patients who are naïve to opioid agonist therapy and do not have contradictions to this medication, because converting from methadone to buprenorphine is difficult and often unsuccessful.

For both patients and providers, it is tempting to choose an agonist therapy or medication-assisted withdrawal based on newborn risks such as NOWS, but we would caution against this practice. There are data to support that buprenorphine maintenance leads to better newborn outcomes. In the only randomized, controlled trial comparing methadone and buprenorphine for the treatment of perinatal OUD, neonates whose mothers were on buprenorphine maintenance therapy, as opposed to methadone maintenance, needed 89% less morphine for NOWS treatment and spent 43% less time (7.5 days) in the hospital.[42] However, first choosing a treatment that will assist pregnant women remain abstinent from drug use will ultimately produce the best outcomes for mothers and their newborns.

There may be opportunities to decrease the potential severity of newborn withdrawal by addressing the use of tobacco and/or concomitant medications, as well as by encouraging breastfeeding. The risk of neonatal opioid withdrawal syndrome increases with the concomitant use of other medications such as gabapentin, benzodiazepines, and antidepressants.[43,44] Cigarette smoking is also associated with more morphine needed to treat neonatal opioid withdrawal syndrome, number of days on medications for neonatal opioid withdrawal syndrome, and a longer duration of hospital stay.[45] Jones and colleagues[45] demonstrated that breastfeeding decreases the severity of neonatal opioid withdrawal syndrome scores, delays the onset of withdrawal and need for medication, and results in shorter hospital durations of stay compared with formula-fed infants. Maternal passage of a small amount of opioid medication to the newborn via breast milk may contribute to the reduced severity of

NOWS. The physical contact and mother–infant bonding associated breastfeeding however may also help to decrease newborn arousal and NOWS symptoms.

Unfortunately, the eligibility of patients for treatment with methadone or buprenorphine relies heavily on the availability of methadone treatment centers or buprenorphine community providers. Although methadone is dispensed at federally designated clinics, buprenorphine is prescribed in the outpatient setting by providers who have completed a buprenorphine waiver training course. Suboxone.com is a valuable resource for identifying buprenorphine prescribers in any community and buprenorphine waiver courses are available through national organizations to physicians in all specialties and to nurse practitioners who are working with a physician who has a buprenorphine license.

Medication-Assisted Withdrawal

Opioid agonist therapy is the standard of care for pregnant women with Opioid Use Disorder and current data do not support the practice of Medication Assisted Withdrawal. However, some women may not have access to opioid agonist therapy and/or may choose to not take this medication during pregnancy. The providers goal is to support women in making an informed treatment choice that is best for her. Pregnant women without a recent or current history of heroin use or intravenous drug use who appreciate the risks for relapse with discontinuation of opioid agonist therapy and continue to express a strong desire to discontinue opioid agonist therapy are potentially good candidates for medication-assisted withdrawal. Other factors that may increase the success of medication-assisted withdrawal include a history of drug abstinence without the use of methadone or buprenorphine, positive social supports, employment, few psychosocial stressors, and a willingness to engage in frequent follow-up appointments and relapse prevention therapy. Any history of relapse to opioid use when previously attempting to taper opioid agonist therapy suggests a high risk for future relapse and, therefore, a medication-assisted taper would not be recommended.

Once a decision is made to start opioid agonist therapy or medication-assisted withdrawal, patients and providers should continue to reevaluate this decision throughout pregnancy. If a woman undergoing medication-assisted withdrawal continues to experience withdrawal symptoms, cravings, or cannot maintain sobriety from opioids, she should begin opioid agonist therapy. Likewise, women who are unsuccessful in abstaining from opioid use with buprenorphine are good candidates for switching to methadone.

Earlier studies examining medication-assisted withdrawal in pregnant women with OUD suggest that there may be an increased risk for poor obstetric outcomes, including intrauterine fetal demise and preterm birth.[29–31,33] Recent studies, however, do not support this association[37–41] and the findings associated with earlier studies are likely owing to relapse to drug use during pregnancy, as opposed to the effects of medication-assisted withdrawal.[29,30,33] There is significant variability in the protocols used to taper opioid medications during pregnancy,[37] but longer tapers with more intensive follow-up care seem to be the most successful in helping women wean opioid medications during pregnancy (**Table 4**).

Patient–physician agreement forms can be used with women who are beginning treatment for OUD and contain statements that ensure patients comprehend their role and responsibilities regarding their treatment. These forms outline the conditions under which treatment may be provided and the responsibilities of the patient and their health care provider. This tool can help to establish boundaries and plans, including protocols for positive UDS and/or other aberrant behavior. These

Table 4
Methadone or buprenorphine medication tapering regimens

Author	Taper Schedule
Lund et al,[40] 2012	7-Day methadone taper All participants (n = 8) were taking methadone 40 mg on day 1 and the dose was lowered to 30 mg on day 2. methadone dose was then reduced by 5 mg each day over 5 d.
Stewart et al,[39] 2013	Gradual methadone taper: Methadone dose was decreased for all participants (n = 95) by no more than 20% of the initial starting dose every 1–3 d as tolerated, until methadone was discontinued. Women with longer tapers were more likely to remain abstinent from opioid use at delivery compared with women who relapsed to opioid use (median 25 d vs 15 d).
Dooley et al,[41] 2015	Gradual morphine or controlled relapse morphine (MS Contin or M-Eslon) taper: Tapering schedule for all participants (n = 86) was described as gradual over months (ie, taper was initiated in the first trimester and completed during the second trimester).
Welle-Strand et al,[38] 2015	Gradual methadone taper Tapering schedule for all participants (n = 123) was described only as a 50% or 10% decrease in methadone dose.
Bell et al,[37] 2016	Variable buprenorphine tapers (1) Abrupt cessation with symptomatic treatment was provided to incarcerated women (n = 108); (2) participants (n = 100) took part in a 5- to 10-d inpatient buprenorphine-assisted withdrawal protocol; and (3) participants (n = 93) completed a 6- to 12-wk outpatient buprenorphine-assisted withdrawal protocol. Rates of relapse to opioid use was lower with intensive follow-up care, compared with no follow-up care (17% vs 74%, respectively).

agreements may serve as a guide to mitigate issues that arise during treatment. Sample forms are widely available for reference if providers do not routinely use these already.[46]

SUMMARY

Obstetricians play a unique and critically important role in the management of perinatal OUD. By using a nonjudgmental approach and discussing the risks and benefits of the available treatment options in general, and for the individual patient, they can help women choose a treatment approach that is best for them. Future research is greatly needed to determine the characteristics of those who are the best candidates for opioid agonist therapy or medication assisted withdrawal. For now, we need to support women in making an informed choice based on limited data and limited perinatal OUD treatment resources. Treatment choice should support patients' values and preferences and ideally have the lowest risk for relapse to drug use to have the most positive impact on maternal and newborn health.

REFERENCES

1. Bateman BT, Hernandez-Diaz S, Rathmell JP, et al. Patterns of opioid utilization in pregnancy in a large cohort of commercial insurance beneficiaries in the United States. Anesthesiology 2014;120(5):1216–24. Available at: http://anesthesiology.pubs.asahq.org/article.aspx?articleid=1917773. Accessed December 15, 2017.

2. Desai RJ, Hernandez-Diaz S, Bateman BT, et al. Increase in prescription opioid use during pregnancy among medicaid-enrolled women. Obstet Gynecol 2014; 123(5):997–1002.

3. Maeda A, Bateman BT, Clancy CR, et al. Opioid abuse and dependence during pregnancy: temporal trends and obstetrical outcomes. Anesthesiology 2014; 121(6):1158–65.

4. Patrick SW, Schumacher RE, Benneyworth BD, et al. Neonatal abstinence syndrome and associated health care expenditures in the united states, 2000-2009. JAMA 2012;307(18):1934–40.

5. Saia K, Schiff D, Wachman E, et al. Caring for pregnant women with opioid use disorder in the USA: expanding and improving treatment. Curr Obstet Gynecol Rep 2016;5:257–63.

6. Guttmacher Institute. Substance abuse during pregnancy. state policies in brief. 2015. Available at: www.guttmacher.org/statecenter/spibs/spib_SADP.pdf. Accessed September 25, 2017.

7. Terplan M, Kennedy-Hendricks A, Chisolm M. Prenatal substance use: exploring assumptions of maternal unfitness. Subst Abuse 2015;9:1–4.

8. ACOG Committee on Health Care for Underserved Women. Committee opinion no. 633: alcohol abuse and other substance use disorders: ethical issues in obstetric and gynecologic practice. Obstet Gynecol 2015;125(6):1529–37. Available at: https://www.acog.org/-/media/Committee-Opinions/Committee-on-Ethics/co633.pdf?d. Accessed September 25, 2017.

9. ACOG Committee on Health Care for Underserved Women; American Society of Addiction Medicine. ACOG committee opinion no. 524: opioid abuse, dependence, and addiction in pregnancy. Obstet Gynecol 2012;119(5):1070–6.

10. World Health Organization: World health statistics 2014. Geneva (Switzerland): WHO; 2014. p. 7–177.

11. Substance Abuse and Mental Health Services Administration (SAMHSA). Results from the 2012 national survey on drug use and health: summary of national findings. 2013. Updated NSDUH Series H-46, HHS Publication No. (SMA) 13–4795. Available at: http://www.samhsa.gov/data/. Accessed December 8, 2017.

12. Klaman SL, Isaacs K, Leopold A, et al. Treating women who are pregnant and parenting for opioid use disorder and the concurrent care of their infants and children: literature review to support national guidance. J Addict Med 2017;11(3): 178–90. Available at: https://www.ncbi.nlm.nih.gov/pmc/articles/PMC5457836/. Accessed December 8, 2017.

13. Wright T, Terplan M, Ondersma S, et al. The role of screening, brief intervention, and referral to treatment in the perinatal period. Am J Obstet Gynecol 2016; 215(5):539–47.

14. Chasnoff IJ, Wells AM, McGourty RF, et al. Validation of the 4P's plus© screen for substance use in pregnancy validation of the 4P's plus. J Perinatol 2007; 27(12):744–8. Available at: https://www.nature.com/articles/7211823. Accessed December 7, 2017.

15. American Society of Addiction Medicine. Public policy statement on substance use, misuse, and use disorders during and following pregnancy, with an emphasis on opioids. ASAM 2017;1–6. Available at: https://www.asam.org/docs/default-source/public-policy-statements/substance-use-misuse-and-use-disorders-during-and-following-pregnancy.pdf?sfvrsn=644978c2_4.

16. Phillips D, Thomas K, Cox Hea. Factors that influence women's disclosures of substance use during pregnancy: a qualitative study of ten midwives and ten pregnant women. J Drug Issues 2007;37(2):357–357-375.

17. American Psychiatric Association. Diagnostic and statistical manual of mental disorders. 5th edition. Arlington (VA): American Psychiatric Association; 2013.

18. Reisfield GM, Webb FJ, Bertholf RL, et al. Family physicians' proficiency in urine drug test interpretation. J Opioid Manag 2007;3(6):333–7. Available at: https://www.researchgate.net/profile/Fern_Webb/publication/5560788_Family_physicians'_proficiency_in_urine_drug_test_interpretation/links/581207a208ae1625bc611e80.pdf. Accessed December 6, 2017.

19. Levy S, Harris SK, Sherritt L, et al. Drug testing of adolescents in ambulatory medicine: physician practices and knowledge. Arch Pediatr Adolesc Med 2006;160(2):146–50.

20. Durback LF, Scharman EJ, Brown BS. Emergency physicians perceptions of drug screens at their own hospitals. Vet Hum Toxicol 1998;40(4):234–7.

21. Dunn KE, Sigmon SC, McGee MR, et al. Evaluation of ongoing oxycodone abuse among methadone-maintained patients. J Subst Abuse Treat 2008;35(4):451–6.

22. Tenore PL. Advanced urine toxicology testing. J Addict Dis 2010;29(4):436–48. Available at: https://www.tandfonline.com/doi/abs/10.1080/10550887.2010.509277. Accessed December 6, 2017.

23. Pavlic M, Libiseller K, Grubwieser P, et al. Cross-reactivity of the CEDIA buprenorphine assay with opiates : an Austrian phenomenon? Int J Legal Med 2005;119:378–81.

24. Saitman A, Hyung-Doo P, Fitgerald R. False-positive interferences of common urine drug screen immunoassays: a review. J Anal Toxicol 2014;38:387–96.

25. Moeller KE, Lee KC, Kissack JC. Urine drug screening: practical guide for clinicians. Mayo Clin Proc 2008;83(1):66–76. Available at: https://www.sciencedirect.com/science/article/pii/S0025619616308254. Accessed December 7, 2017.

26. Schuckit MA. Treatment of opioid-use disorders. N Engl J Med 2016;375(4):357–68.

27. Kampman K, Jarvis M. American society of addiction medicine (ASAM) national practice guideline for the use of medications in the treatment of addiction involving opioid use. J Addict Med 2015;9(5):358–67. Available at: https://www.ncbi.nlm.nih.gov/pmc/articles/PMC4605275/. Accessed December 18, 2017.

28. Substance Abuse and Mental Health Services Administration (SAMHSA). Center for Substance Abuse Treatment. Substance abuse treatment: addressing the specific needs of women. Treatment improvement protocol (TIP) series, no. 51. HHS publication no. (SMA) 15-4426. Rockville (MD): Center for Substance Abuse Treatment; 2009. Updated HHS Publication No. (SMA) 15-4426. Available at: https://store.samhsa.gov/shin/content/SMA15-4426/SMA15-4426.pdf.

29. Maas U, Kattner E, Weingart-Jesse B, et al. Infrequent neonatal opiate withdrawal following maternal methadone detoxification during pregnancy. J Perinat Med 1990;18(2):111–8. Available at: https://www.degruyter.com/dg/viewarticle/j$002fjpme.1990.18.issue-2$002fjpme.1990.18.2.111$002fjpme.1990.18.2.111.xml. Accessed December 18, 2017.

30. Dashe JS, Jackson GL, Olscher DA, et al. Opioid detoxification in pregnancy. Obstet Gynecol 1998;92(5):854–8.

31. Luty J, Nikolaou V, Bearn J. Is opiate detoxification unsafe in pregnancy? J Subst Abuse Treat 2003;24:363–7. Available at: https://www.sciencedirect.com/science/article/pii/S0740547203000357. Accessed December 18, 2017.

32. Jones HE, O'Grady KE, Malfi D, et al. Methadone maintenance vs. methadone taper during pregnancy: maternal and neonatal outcomes. Am J Addict 2008;17(5):372–86.

33. Blinick G, Wallach RC, Jerez E, et al. Drug addiction in pregnancy and the neonate. Am J Obstet Gynecol 1976;125(2):135–42. Available at: https://www.ajog.org/article/0002-9378(76)90583-4/abstract. Accessed December 18, 2017.
34. Binder T, Vavrinková B. Prospective randomised comparative study of the effect of buprenorphine, methadone and heroin on the course of pregnancy, birthweight of newborns, early postpartum adaptation and course of the neonatal abstinence syndrome (NAS) in women followed up in the outpatient department. Neuro Endocrinol Lett 2008;29(1):80–6. Available at: https://europepmc.org/abstract/med/18283247. Accessed December 6, 2017.
35. McCarthy JJ, Leamon MH, Parr MS, et al. High-dose methadone maintenance in pregnancy: maternal and neonatal outcomes. Am J Obstet Gynecol 2005;193(3):606–10.
36. Sigmon SC. Characterizing the emerging population of prescription opioid abusers. Am J Addict 2006;15(3):208–12. Available at: https://onlinelibrary.wiley.com/doi/abs/10.1080/10550490600625624. Accessed December 6, 2017.
37. Bell J, Towers CV, Hennessy MD, et al. Detoxification from opiate drugs during pregnancy. Am J Obstet Gynecol 2016;215(3):374.e1-6.
38. Welle-Strand GK, Skurtveit S, Tanum L, et al. Tapering from methadone or buprenorphine during pregnancy: maternal and neonatal outcomes in Norway 1996-2009. Eur Addict Res 2015;21(5):253–61.
39. Stewart RD, Nelson DB, Adhikari EH, et al. The obstetrical and neonatal impact of maternal opioid detoxification in pregnancy. Am J Obstet Gynecol 2013;209(3):267.e1-5.
40. Lund IO, Fitzsimons H, Tuten M, et al. Comparing methadone and buprenorphine maintenance with methadone-assisted withdrawal for the treatment of opioid dependence during pregnancy: maternal and neonatal outcomes. Subst Abuse Rehabil 2012;3:17–25.
41. Dooley R, Dooley J, Antone I, et al. Narcotic tapering in pregnancy using long-acting morphine: an 18-month prospective cohort study in northwestern Ontario. Can Fam Physician 2015;61(2):e88–95.
42. Jones HE, Kaltenbach K, Heil SH. Neonatal abstinence syndrome after methadone or buprenorphine exposure. N Engl J Med 2010;363(24):2320–31.
43. Huybrechts KF, Bateman BT, Desai RJ, et al. Risk of neonatal drug withdrawal after intrauterine co-exposure to opioids and psychotropic medications: cohort study. BMJ 2017;358. Available at: https://www.bmj.com/content/358/bmj.j3326. Accessed December 6, 2017.
44. Patrick SW, Cooper WO, Davis MM. Prescribing opioids and psychotropic drugs in pregnancy. BMJ 2017;358. Available at: https://www.bmj.com/content/358/bmj.j3616.full. Accessed December 6, 2017.
45. Jones HE, Heil SH, Tuten M, et al. Cigarette smoking in opioid-dependent pregnant women: neonatal and maternal outcomes. Drug Alcohol Depend 2013;131(3):271–7.
46. National Institute on Drug Abuse. Sample patient agreement forms. Available at: https://www.drugabuse.gov/sites/default/files/files/SamplePatientAgreementForms.pdf. Accessed December 6, 2017.

Impact of Pregnancy Loss on Psychological Functioning and Grief Outcomes

Tonia M. Cassaday, MSW, LISW-CP/S

KEYWORDS

- Perinatal loss • Perinatal grief • Perinatal bereavement • Psychological functioning

KEY POINTS

- Perinatal grief is a common and natural occurrence. When parents cannot seem to work through the common grief reactions, complicated grief may become evident. Risk factors and treatment of complicated grief are discussed.
- Mothers and fathers often have different reactions to perinatal loss and grieve in different ways. The gender differences in the grieving process are discussed, as well as the impact of grief on relationships.
- Health care professionals are in an important position to make a positive difference for parents who are grieving a perinatal loss. The role of the professional is discussed, including screening and treatment of perinatal loss.

INTRODUCTION

Stillbirth is defined as the death of a fetus after 20 weeks gestation with a birthweight of more than 500 g. Miscarriage is generally defined as an unintended termination of pregnancy before 20 weeks of gestation. In contrast, pregnancy termination is usually a planned event following a diagnosis of fetal abnormality.[1] Perinatal loss is the nonvoluntary end of pregnancy or death of the baby from conception until 28 days into a newborn's life. The term perinatal loss includes miscarriage, stillbirth, and neonatal death.[2]

The loss of a child is associated with a grief experience that is particularly severe, long-lasting, and complicated, with symptoms that fluctuate in intensity and duration.[3] Grief symptoms of perinatal loss are usually processed in stages and decrease in intensity over time. These symptoms often decline significantly by 6 months for

Disclosure Statement: This author has no relationship with a commercial company that has a direct financial interest in the subject matter or materials discussed in this article or with a company making a competing product.
Department of Psychiatry, Medical University of South Carolina, 65 President Street, Charleston, SC 29425, USA
E-mail address: cassaday@musc.edu

Obstet Gynecol Clin N Am 45 (2018) 525–533
https://doi.org/10.1016/j.ogc.2018.04.004
0889-8545/18/© 2018 Elsevier Inc. All rights reserved.

obgyn.theclinics.com

both men and women. Though there is no order or time limit associated with the reactions, the grief process is usually 12 to 24 months with symptoms lessening over time.

Based on a review of literature, this article describes the prevalence, timing, and common reactions to perinatal grief and loss. The aim is to help obstetricians differentiate between uncomplicated and complicated grief, as well as recognize the factors that may increase the risk for complicated grief following perinatal loss. Gender differences and the impact of perinatal loss on relationships is highlighted. Finally, the article provides guidance for the obstetrician working with bereaved parents, including recommendations for screening and evidence-based treatments.

PREVALENCE AND TIMING OF PERINATAL LOSS

In 2007, the infant mortality rate in the United States was 6.9 deaths per 1000 live births. The overall prevalence for miscarriage is 15% to 27% for women aged between 25 and 29 years, and 75% in women older than 45 years. The risk of miscarriage is even higher in women with prior pregnancy loss.[1]

Of an estimated 6,578,000 pregnancies in the United States in 2008, almost one-fifth (1,118,000 or 17%) resulted in documented fetal losses. The actual rate is much higher, however, because many women have very early miscarriages without ever realizing that they were pregnant.[4–6] Of women who experience perinatal loss, 50% to 80% become pregnant again.[2]

According to the Centers for Disease Control and Prevention, stillbirth affects about 1% of all pregnancies. Each year about 24,000 babies are stillborn in the United States. This is about the same number of babies who die during the first year of life and it is more than 10 times as many deaths as the number that occurs from sudden infant death syndrome. Because of advances in medical technology over the last 30 years, prenatal care has improved, which has dramatically reduced the number of late and term stillbirths. The rate of early stillbirth, however, has remained about the same over time. Although stillbirth occurs in families of all races, ethnicities, and income levels, and to women of all ages, some women are at higher risk for having a stillbirth. Some of the factors that increase the risk for a stillbirth include:

- African-American race
- Teenager
- 35 years of age or older
- Unmarried
- Obese
- Smoking cigarettes during pregnancy
- Medical conditions, such as high blood pressure or diabetes
- Multiple pregnancies
- Previous pregnancy loss.[7]

A study by Theut and colleagues[8] revealed that the nature and intensity of the grief experienced by the parents is different when the loss occurs later in pregnancy. This difference may be related to the intensity of the physical and emotional attachment, which in turn is related to the duration of the pregnancy. For example, later in the pregnancy, the parents will have noticed the physical changes of the mother's body, felt the baby's movement, heard the fetal heartbeat, and viewed ultrasound pictures. Thus, for both parents, the baby would have become increasingly real.

COMMON GRIEF REACTIONS

Initial common reactions to the loss of a fetus are often shock, disbelief, and numbness. The reality of the loss may be denied to avoid the pain. These reactions provide emotional protection from being overwhelmed emotionally all at once. Once the shock begins to fade, it is often replaced with unbearable pain. Although this grief reaction is excruciating, it is important that bereaved parents experience their pain fully. Avoidance of the pain associated with perinatal loss during the grief process can lead to negative coping mechanisms such as alcohol or drugs to numb the pain. The parents may also experience guilt or remorse at this time about things that they did or did not do during the pregnancy. The pain and guilt often give way to anger. During this grief reaction, bereaved parents may lash out at medical providers or lay unwarranted blame on others or even each other. This reaction is dangerous because it can result in permanent damage to and lasting effects on relationships. During this reaction, parents may also protest vehemently against fate and question it. They may bargain in vain with the powers that be for a way out of their despair. The next grief reaction is a long period of sadness, loneliness, isolation, emptiness, despair, and self-reflection. This reaction usually takes places months after the loss has occurred. It is during this time that grieving parents realize the true impact of their loss. Next, parents begin to adjust to life without their baby and their lives become a little calmer and more controlled. Their physical symptoms improve and their sadness begins to lift slightly. As they become more functioning, bereaved parents find themselves making realistic and sound solutions to life's problems and reconstructing their lives without their baby. It is also during this reaction that parents learn to accept and deal with the loss of their child. They find a way to move forward with their lives. They make plans for the future and look forward to experiencing them. In time, they remember their baby without pain and find joy in life again. A valuable patient and provider resource describing the stages of grief can be found at www.recover-from-grief.com/7stages-of-grief.

It is important to mention that these grief reactions must be interpreted loosely. There is not an orderly progression from reaction to reaction. The progression varies among individuals and there is no time limit on grief. The events surrounding the death, as well as past experiences of loss, have an impact on the individual grieving process. Some parents get back to their routine fairly quickly and others take longer. Some parents prefer time alone to grieve and others crave the support and company of others. These grief reactions are simply a guide of what to expect.

COMPLICATED GRIEF AND RISK FACTORS

Although grief is a natural, nonpathologic phenomenon, it can lead to complicated grief in which symptoms are more disruptive or long-lasting.[4] Complicated grief is a term used to describe when people adjust poorly to a loss. Based on clinical experience, complicated grief is more likely to occur if the death occurred suddenly, violently, or traumatically, which is often the case in perinatal loss. **Box 1** lists some warning signs that may suggest that a person is not coping well with grief and may be at a greater risk of the grieving process taking longer to resolve or being more difficult.

Perinatal loss leads to complicated grief more frequently than other losses. This loss represents not only a physical absence but also a psychological presence, especially for the mother who carried the baby in her womb before its death.[3] Several factors that may contribute to complicated grief are:

- The loss is often sudden and unexpected
- The loss is often not openly acknowledged

Box 1
Warning signs of complicated grief

- Pushing away painful feelings or avoiding the grieving process entirely
- Excessive avoidance of talking about or reminders of the baby that died
- Refusal to plan and/or attend a funeral (if appropriate)
- Using distracting tasks to avoid experiencing grief
- Abuse of alcohol or drugs, including prescription drugs
- Increased physical complaints or illness
- Intense mood swings or isolation that do not resolve within 1 to 2 months
- Ongoing neglect of self-care and responsibilities at home, school, or work

Adapted from Centre for Clinical Interventions. Grief and bereavement 2016. Available at: http://www.cci.health.wa.gov.au/docs/ACF3185.pdf. Accessed August 31, 2017; with permission.

- The loss is often not socially supported
- The loss is associated with guilt or self-blame
- There are no memories or experiences to share
- There is no concrete object to mourn.[2,4]

Despite many studies on the risk factors of grief, little prospective research documents what parents undergo after any type of perinatal loss. Little has been published on the association of grief and perinatal loss, thus few clear and consistent results are evident.[4] The risk factors for complicated grief are believed to include:

- Young maternal age
- Decreased social supports
- Recurrent pregnancy loss
- History of trauma
- Preexisting psychiatric illness
- Having no living children
- A longer pregnancy
- A history of infertility
- Having no religious beliefs
- Not having participated in rituals for the deceased baby
- Having low marriage satisfaction
- Preexisting relationship difficulties.[2,4]

GENDER DIFFERENCES AND IMPACT ON RELATIONSHIPS

The mother–baby relationship is unique. Very early on in the pregnancy, the mother forms a bond with the baby. The baby actually becomes part of the mother's body and the mother becomes "invested by her as a part of the self."[8] For the father, the relationship to the baby is always more mental. Thus, the mother–baby relationship is different than the father–baby relationship. The bereavement of the mother for the loss of a child is unique in that she is grieving for loss of a part of herself. For the father, the attachment from the beginning is different and the resulting bereavement is thought to be different.[8]

According to Bhat and Byatt,[2] findings of a few small studies indicate that there seems to be a lower rate of distress in men compared with women after perinatal loss. Men may also grieve differently, preferring to talk less, present as irritable, and have heavier alcohol consumption. In addition, men seem to grieve less intensively and for shorter periods than their partners do.

Symptoms of grieving in men were found to be similar to those of women, except that men report less crying and feel less need to talk about their loss.[1] Depressive symptoms for men after a perinatal loss is greater within the first month (5%–17%), then decreases to 7% at 3 months and 1% to 4% at 6 months.[2] In general, the longer the pregnancy, the more intense is the grief in men.[9]

In addition to a grieving mother blaming herself, she may place blame on the father and he is often the target of the mother's anger. This can happen because the mother blames him for not having the same feelings that she has, or at least she perceives that they are not the same. Generally, in the circumstances surrounding perinatal loss, the father feels powerless and his need to act strong and to be supportive may be misinterpreted by the mother as not caring.[9] Fathers have reported feeling ignored and unacknowledged as a legitimately grieving parent due to the mothers being the main focus during perinatal loss.[3] One of the greatest challenges for the father is to provide support for their partner while trying to cope with grief himself.

Within couples, partners have different expectations about how to react, how to behave, and what is an appropriate length of time to grieve. For the couples themselves, misunderstandings and divergent perceptions about the meaning of the loss and about the right way to grieve also sometimes creates an emotional distance between them. The experience of perinatal loss can alter how parents feel about themselves and each other.[3] A study by Theut and colleagues[8] in 1989 revealed that couples who experience either early or late loss grieve less after the birth of a viable child.

ROLE OF THE HEALTH CARE PROFESSIONAL

Health care providers in perinatal settings may encounter death infrequently and, as a result, often feel inadequately prepared to take care of families when death occurs.[10] Although the care provided to parents after a perinatal loss varies, parents want medical staff to be sensitive and empathic to their needs. They want their feelings validated and, if possible, clear information about what happened and why, and about how, where, and when they can meaningfully express their grief.[4] Even though this information can be helpful to the grieving parents, it is also important that the medical staff recognize that they have sustained a significant loss and not try to mask or minimize the loss with an upbeat focus on the future and the possibility of future pregnancies. Future pregnancies are certainly a concern of the parents but many health professionals, in their discomfort about a perinatal loss, may deal with this by focusing on this issue alone.[9]

A 2011 study by Lang and colleagues[3] revealed that health care professionals hold an advantageous position to assist grieving parents with the effects of perinatal loss, yet studies suggest that their impact in this regard can be inadequate or even hurtful. Their lack of knowledge about the physical, emotional, and social impact of perinatal loss on individuals and families, together with a sense of discomfort with bereavement and how to attend to the bereaved, frequently spills over into care provision. Rather than assisting, health care professionals can often intensify parental grief when they fail to recognize how their actions, comments, and behaviors affect the experiences of their vulnerable patients. Comforting words of kindness and touch have the potential to have long-lasting healing effects but callousness and indifference (often unintentional) can severely compound an already difficult experience for the grieving parents. It has been reported that, more often than not, bereaved parents receive inappropriate or insensitive care following a perinatal death, even though there are well-accepted standards of care that exist in the theoretic and research literature, as well as among professionals in the field.

Health care professionals need to be sensitive to and aware of their contribution to bereaved parents' distress surrounding perinatal loss. These vulnerable parents are often hypersensitive to every look, touch, comment, or reaction by health care providers. Regardless of whether such interactions are perceived by the parents as supportive or hurtful, they are filed in their memory forever and this will color their bereavement experience and how they cope with the death of their baby. There is great potential for significantly easing the burdens of these experiences through direct interactions with bereaved couples by conveying empathy, information, and guidance regarding what to expect physically, emotionally, and socially.[3]

The process for health care professionals to assist grieving parents (**Table 1**) can be broken down into 5 steps:

1. Communicate complete sensitivity and empathy.
2. Have a working knowledge of common grief reactions, stages of bereavement, and signs or symptoms of complicated grief.

Table 1
Common symptoms of grief and recommendations for care

Presenting Signs or Symptoms	Care Plan
Common symptoms of uncomplicated grief 　Poor sleep 　Lowered appetite 　Low mood 　Feelings of anxiety 　Sense of loss 　Refusal to believe loss has occurred 　Feeling disconnected from others 　Sense of numbness 　Feelings of guilt 　Worries about not grieving correctly 　Mood swings 　Tearfulness 　Waves of sadness or anger 　Feeling overwhelmed 　Seeking reminders 　Feeling that you see or hear the deceased 　　person 　Guilt about gradually getting back to 　　normal life 　Isolation	Provider recommendation for care 　Most parents experiencing uncomplicated grief will not require medication or psychotherapy. These parents will simply need to go through the natural grieving process and, in time, will adjust to the loss and return to their normal life. It is important, however, that parents reach out to their supports and maintain a healthy lifestyle during the grieving process. Some parents, however, do benefit from psychotherapy and/or support groups during this time.
Common symptoms of complicated grief 　Pushing away painful feelings 　Avoidance of the grief process 　Refusal to attend the funeral (if applicable) 　Abuse of alcohol or other drug 　Increase in physical complaints or illness 　Intense mood swings 　Prolonged isolation 　Neglect of self-care 　Neglect of responsibilities at home or work	Provider recommendation for care 　Psychotherapy can assist parents to safely explore their grief reactions and pave the way for resolution. Medication may also be prescribed to alleviate the depressive and anxious symptoms associated with complicated grief. Early intervention is best but progress can be made long after the loss occurs.

Data from Centre for Clinical Interventions. Grief and bereavement 2016. Available at: http://www.cci.health.wa.gov.au/docs/ACF3185.pdf. Accessed August 31, 2017.

3. Be familiar with your clinic's protocols regarding bereavement.
4. Be aware of the family's needs and make appropriate referrals.
5. Follow-up with the family to ensure that their needs are being met.

The following are comments that health care professional should avoid when working with bereaved parents:

- You can always have another child.
- At least you have other children.
- You are young and have plenty of time.
- It's better that it happened now rather than later when you have bonded with your child.
- This is a blessing, things probably would have been worse of it had not happened now.
- This is simply nature's way.
- You can use the items you have purchased for the next baby.

SCREENING AND TREATMENT

Even though 30% of women report that they would have liked to discuss the causes of their miscarriage and the risk for future pregnancies, 90% do not receive a follow-up visit with their provider to allow for this discussion. Ideally, a screening would take place 6 weeks following the perinatal loss as women's responses at the 6 weeks marker have been shown to predict their responses at the 1 year marker. Common screening instruments include:

- Perinatal Grief Scale
- The Munich Grief Scale
- The Perinatal Bereavement Scale
- Perinatal Grief Intensity Scale
- The Dyadic Adjustment Scale
- Impact of Event Scale.[2,4]

Screening, psychoeducation, provision of resources and referrals, and an opportunity to discuss their loss and plan for future pregnancies can facilitate addressing mental health concerns that arise. Women at risk of or who are currently experiencing psychiatric symptoms should receive a comprehensive treatment plan that includes:

1. Proactive clinical monitoring
2. Evidence-based approaches to psychotherapy
3. Discussion of the risks and benefits of, and alternatives to, medication treatment during preconception and pregnancy.[2]

Psychotherapy can support bereaved parents in safely exploring their feelings of grief and connecting with painful feelings and memories, paving the way for resolution. Therapy may also support parents in using strategies such as relaxation, engaging in positive activities, and challenging negative thoughts to combat the associated symptoms of anxiety and depression. From clinical experience, cognitive behavioral therapy, interpersonal therapy, and couples therapy work well with this population. Therapy should involve both grieving parents and ensure an ongoing dialogue between them.

The therapist can also make suggestions that help make the loss more tangible and facilitate the expression of grief, such as naming the fetus, having a memorial service in which a candle is lit or a tree is planted, and finding ways to put the hopes and dreams for the infant into words, such as writing a poem or letter to the baby. A meaningful collection of articles related to the baby can also make the loss real.[9]

Medication, such as antidepressants, may also be used to alleviate depression associated with grief, and this can be useful in conjunction with psychotherapy strategies. Though tranquilizers, such as benzodiazepines, may be helpful initially, they carry significant risks and should not be used long-term. Medication should only be prescribed after a detailed discussion regarding the risks and benefits.

Although early intervention is recommended, mental health professionals are able to support parents to work through complicated grief even years after the loss. Other approaches to supporting grieving parents after perinatal loss include:

- Informational and supportive DVDs
- Internet-based cognitive behavioral therapy
- Mindfulness-based therapy
- Physical activity
- Keeping a journal or diary
- Encouraging supports to acknowledge important dates related to the loss.

Attendance to a grief and loss support group can also be very beneficial. Talking with others, especially others who have experienced similar loss can be therapeutic for bereaved parents. Having a platform to share feelings is an integral part of the grieving process.

SUMMARY

Grief following perinatal loss is a common and normal occurrence. Even though most women do not need any type of intervention to deal with the loss, it is important that they be screened and monitored, especially if risk factors are present. It is important for health care professionals to increase their ability to identify the factors that psychologically affect grief.

Recommendations for all grieving parents are accessible interventions that include home-based and Internet-based therapies, as well as space for the bereaved parents to discuss and experience their loss. Recommendations for parents with risk factors include a customized treatment plan that incorporates evidence-based interventions such as psychotherapy and medication management.

Often, parents have already picked out names, furnished the nursery, purchased clothing, and envisioned many activities with their child long before the baby is known to the rest of the world. Reconstructing a life without their baby is certainly the most daunting task of perinatal loss, yet in the midst of this profound grieve personal growth can occur.

REFERENCES

1. Kersting A, Wagner B. Complicated grief after perinatal loss. Dialogues Clin Neurosci 2012;14(2):187–94.
2. Bhat A, Byatt N. Infertility and perinatal loss: when the bough breaks. Curr Psychiatry Rep 2016;18(3):31.
3. Lang A, Fleiszer A, Duhamel F, et al. Perinatal loss and perinatal grief: the challenge of ambiguity and disenfranchised grief. Omega 2011;63(2):183–96.
4. Tseng Y-F, Cheng H-R, Chen Y-P, et al. Grief reactions of couples to perinatal loss: a one-year prospective follow-up. J Clin Nurs 2017;00:1–10.

5. Recover-from-grief. 7 stages of grief: through the process and back to life. 2017. Available at: http://www.recover-from-grief.com/7-stages-of-grief.html. Assessed June 20, 2017.
6. Center for Clinical Interventions. Grief and bereavement. 2016. Available at: https://www.cci.health.wa.gov.au. Accessed August 31, 2017.
7. Centers for Disease Control and Prevention. Facts about stillbirth. 2017. Available at: https://www.cdc.gov/ncbdd/stillbirth/facts.html. Accessed November 28, 2017.
8. Theut S, Pedersen F, Zaslow M, et al. Perinatal loss and perinatal bereavement. Am J Psychiatry 1989;5:146.
9. Worden W. Grieving special types of losses. In: Sussman SW, Rosen J, editors. Grief counseling and grief therapy: a handbook for the mental health practitioner. New York: Springer Publishing Company; 2009. p. 195–7.
10. Black BP, Limbo RK, Wright PM. My absent child: cultural and theoretical consideration of bereavement when a child dies. In: Nieginski E, Exeter Premedia Servcies Private, LTD, editors. Perinatal and pediatric bereavement in nursing and other health professions. New York: Springer Publishing Company; 2015. p. 8–10.

Perinatal Intimate Partner Violence

Christine K. Hahn, PhD*, Amanda K. Gilmore, PhD,
Rosaura Orengo Aguayo, PhD, Alyssa A. Rheingold, PhD

KEYWORDS

- Intimate partner violence • Physical violence • Sexual violence • Perinatal
- Pregnancy

KEY POINTS

- Violence perpetrated by an intimate partner is estimated to occur in 3.7% to 9.0% of perinatal women.
- There is a pervasive impact of perinatal IPV on several psychological and physical outcomes relevant to the mother and child. These include grave outcomes, such as suicidal ideation, stillbirths, and maternal death.
- Screening for IPV during perinatal health care visits is essential to detect women who are at risk for adverse obstetric health outcomes, facilitate safety planning, and initiate referral to mental health treatment.

Intimate partner violence (IPV) is a serious public health problem that involves physical violence, sexual violence, stalking, psychological aggression, or control of reproductive health perpetrated by a current or former intimate partner (**Box 1**).[1,2] An intimate partner is an individual with whom one has a close personal relationship; however, the characteristics of the relationship, such the degree of contact or familiarity with one another can vary.[1] Based on results from the National Intimate Partner and Sexual Violence Survey, 5.9% of women reported experiencing IPV in the past year.[2] Prevalence of lifetime exposure to specific forms of IPV is alarming, ranging from 8.6% for reproductive control to 47.1% for psychological aggression.

The highest rates of IPV are reported among women who are of reproductive age, with the greatest prevalence occurring among individuals 18 to 34 years old.[1,2]

Disclosure Statement: The authors do not have any commercial or financial conflicts of interests. Authors do not have any funding that is supporting this article. This work was supported by the [National Institute of Mental Health] under Grant [T32MHH018869].
Department of Psychiatry and Behavioral Sciences, Medical University of South Carolina, National Crime Victims Research and Treatment Center (NCVRTC), 67 President Street, 2nd Floor South, MSC 861, Charleston, SC 29425-8610, USA
* Corresponding author.
E-mail address: hahnc@musc.edu

Obstet Gynecol Clin N Am 45 (2018) 535–547
https://doi.org/10.1016/j.ogc.2018.04.008
0889-8545/18/© 2018 Elsevier Inc. All rights reserved.

obgyn.theclinics.com

Box 1
Definitions and lifetime prevalence of forms of intimate partner violence

Physical Violence (32.4%)
- Behaviors with the potential for causing injury, harm, disability, or death
- Examples include slapping, pushing, choking, pulling hair, kicking, and use of restraint

Sexual Violence (16.4%)
- Unwanted sexual experiences that range from noncontact to completed rape
- Rape includes completed forced penetration, attempted forced penetration, and completed alcohol or drug-facilitated penetration

Stalking (27.4%)
- Patterns of harassing or threating tactics that cause fear or safety concerns

Psychological Aggression (47.1%)
- Expressive aggression and coercive control behaviors
- Examples include name-calling, insults, denying access to basic resources

Control of Reproductive or Sexual Health (8.6%)
- Refusal to wear a condom or attempting to get a person pregnant when the person did not want to become pregnant

---

Therefore, it is essential to investigate IPV among perinatal women. The current review outlines the following for IPV:

1. Definition and prevalence
2. Maternal risk factors and obstetric health associations
3. Neonatal outcomes
4. Long-term impact on children
5. Screening and referral interventions

PERINATAL INTIMATE PARTNER VIOLENCE

Perinatal IPV refers to experiences of violence that occur 12 months before pregnancy, during pregnancy, and up to 1 year following a pregnancy.[3,4] Based on population studies, estimated rates of perinatal IPV in the form of physical violence range from 3.7% to 9.0%.[3,4] However, it is difficult to estimate the rates of perinatal IPV because these population-based studies have focused on physical violence, without adequately assessing for other forms of perinatal IPV, such as sexual violence and psychological aggression. Further, frequencies of IPV are higher in clinic-based samples compared with epidemiologic samples. Among 104 rural women attending prenatal care in the beginning of their third trimester, 20.2% experienced sexual IPV, 27.9% reported physical IPV, and 79.8% endorsed psychological aggression during their pregnancy.[5] Other clinic-based studies have reported rates of perinatal IPV up to 16.4% and 73.0% for physical and psychological IPV, respectively.[6,7] Perinatal providers are in a unique position to identify, evaluate, and facilitate services for women experiencing IPV.

MATERNAL RISK FACTORS AND MENTAL AND OBSTETRIC HEALTH ASSOCIATIONS OF PERINATAL INTIMATE PARTNER VIOLENCE

Risk factors for perinatal IPV include lower socioeconomic status, being unmarried, housing instability, younger age, Medicaid insurance, and fewer years of education.[4,8] Rates of IPV tend to be slightly higher during the year before pregnancy than during pregnancy. For example, based on data from the Pregnancy Risk Assessment Monitoring System, 4.7% of women reported physical violence perpetrated by a partner in the year before pregnancy compared with 3.7% during pregnancy.[4] Exposure to IPV among perinatal women is associated with a host of pervasive and serious maternal mental and physical health consequences.

Mental Health

Perinatal IPV is associated with symptoms of posttraumatic stress disorder (PTSD), major depressive disorder, and problematic substance use, which typically extends to postpartum periods (**Box 2**).[6,9] It is important to distinguish the nature of perinatal IPV from other forms of traumatic events. In population-based studies, women exposed to various forms of interpersonal violence (eg, child abuse, sexual abuse, IPV) have high rates of PTSD, depressive, and substance use symptoms.[10,11] These symptoms are typically higher among individuals exposed to interpersonal violence compared with individuals who have other experiences of traumatic events, such as natural disasters, armed conflicts, or accidents.[11] High rates of symptoms may result from IPV because of contextual factors, such as the relationship with the perpetrator and nature of the abuse. For example, within IPV the perpetrator may be someone who

---

Box 2
Common mental health symptoms among women exposed to intimate partner violence

Posttraumatic stress disorder symptoms develop after exposure to 1 or more traumatic events and are characterized by 4 clusters of symptoms:

- Reexperiencing or intrusive thoughts and memories about the traumatic event and intense reactions to cues that remind the individual of the event.

- Avoidance of external (eg, people or places) and internal cues (eg, feelings or thoughts).

- Changes in one's cognitions and mood, including exaggerated self-blame, and decreased interest in pleasurable activities and ability to experience positive emotions.

- Arousal and reactivity difficulties, such as increased irritability, exaggerated startle response, concentration difficulties, sleep problems, hypervigilance, and reckless behaviors.

Major depressive disorder symptoms are marked by depressed mood and loss of interest or pleasure. Symptoms include the following:

- Changes in weight or appetite
- Sleep disturbance
- Suicidal ideation
- Fatigue
- Worthlessness
- Psychomotor agitation or retardation
- Difficulty concentrating

Substance use disorder symptoms can be in relation to various substances ranging from alcohol to nicotine. Symptoms include the following:

- Impaired control, such as taking the substance longer than intended, cravings, and spending a significant amount of time attempting to get access to, use, or recover from the substance

- Impairment in social functioning or use of the substance in risky situations

- Tolerance or withdrawal from the substance

the individual depends on for emotional, financial, or instrumental (eg, household chores, child care) support. In addition, IPV is invasive, and, more often than not, involves repeated victimizations. Women exposed to IPV often experience ongoing legitimate fear about the potential for future harm, which can exacerbate distress.[12] These contextual factors are especially relevant to risk for developing mental health symptoms.

Perinatal physical, sexual, and psychological IPV are associated with PTSD during and after pregnancy. For instance, 40% of low-income pregnant women who reported perinatal IPV met criteria for PTSD.[13] Most of these low-income pregnant women reported that other life events were distressful; therefore, many women with perinatal IPV may have exposure to several traumatic events, which is associated with worse mental health outcomes.[11] Perinatal physical and psychological IPV is also associated with increased depressive symptoms during pregnancy[14] and postpartum.[15] More specifically, among a large urban sample, women who endorsed perinatal IPV were 3 times more likely to meet criteria for depressive disorders during pregnancy.[16] In addition, perinatal IPV was associated with increased risk of depression and PTSD symptoms among women who had delivered their child in the past 14 months.[17] Finally, compared with women who are not exposed to perinatal IPV, women with exposure reported higher levels of suicidal ideation during pregnancy[18] and subsequent to delivery.[19] During 2003 to 2007, 2.0 per 100,000 births resulted in maternal suicide and 54.3% of the people who committed suicide experienced IPV that was suspected to relate to the suicide.[20]

Nicotine, drug, and alcohol use is also a concern among women exposed to perinatal IPV.[21,22] Although many women are able to successfully refrain from using substances while pregnant, the prolonged stress and fear associated with IPV can make abstaining difficult. The self-medication model proposes that substance use is reinforcing because it reduces distress, therefore over time it becomes a pattern of learned behavior to cope with distress.[23] In support of this theory, more severe IPV, PTSD, and depression symptoms predicted greater problems with substance use among community samples of women.[24] With regard to perinatal IPV and nicotine use, physical IPV the year before and/or during pregnancy was associated with a 2.6 times increased risk of smoking cigarettes during pregnancy compared with non-abused women.[25]

Substance use and mental health symptoms also frequently co-occur among women exposed to perinatal IPV. In a primarily Latina sample of pregnant women, those with perinatal IPV and depressive symptoms were more likely to report co-occurring substance use problems.[26] Further, among a sample of women attending prenatal visits, women with positive alcohol use screens were 2.26 more likely to report physical IPV within the past year, and women who had positive depression screens were 3.37 times more likely to report physical IPV in the past year.[27] Taken together, research supports that women who report perinatal IPV are also at increased risk to use alcohol, nicotine, and drugs compared with women who do not report IPV.

In summary, lifetime exposure to IPV and perinatal IPV poses significant risk for women to experience PTSD, depression, suicidal ideation, and use nicotine during perinatal periods.[25,26] Furthermore, IPV 6 to 12 months after delivery results in higher levels of distress and depression compared with women who are not exposed to postpartum violence.[28] Therefore, providers need to be aware that exposure to lifetime IPV may elevate risk for mental health distress among perinatal women. The impact of perinatal IPV moves beyond mental health consequences to a range of obstetric health outcomes.

Obstetric Health

There is substantial evidence that perinatal IPV is linked to multiple obstetric complications. Exposure to IPV may affect women's physical health through direct impact of physical violence that results in maternal or utero-placental injury. However, another mechanism is related to the body's response to acute and chronic stress. The impact of exposure to acute and chronic stress can result in overactive and underactive responses in the hypothalamic-pituitary-adrenal (HPA) axis.[12] The HPA axis regulates hormone secretion through a negative feedback system, which involves interaction between the hypothalamus and pituitary and adrenal glands that communicate signals to reduce or increase the production of hormones, such as cortisol or cortisol-releasing factor. Exposure to IPV can impact the negative feedback system, thereby affecting the secretion of hormones in a manner that can have negative implications for autoimmune and inflammatory responses.

The physiologic impact related to frequent and ongoing threat associated with IPV may be especially relevant to obstetric health. Women who experienced perinatal IPV are more likely to have high blood pressure or edema, vaginal bleeding in the second or third trimester, severe nausea, vomiting or dehydration, kidney infection or urinary tract infection (UTI), premature rupture of membranes, and premature birth.[4] Women with IPV are 5 times more likely to experience placental abruption, or separation of the placenta from the uterus, a complication associated with fetal growth restriction, preterm birth, and intrauterine fetal demise.[8] Regarding timing of perinatal IPV, exposure to IPV before and during pregnancy has been associated with negative health outcomes; however, some risks may become greater for women who experience abuse 12 months before becoming pregnant, including vaginal bleeding, severe nausea, vomiting or dehydration, and kidney infections or UTI.[4]

Perinatal IPV is also associated with miscarriages, preterm birth, and diminished intrauterine growth,[4,29,30] with results from one study supporting that psychological IPV had a greater impact than physical IPV on low birth weight.[30] Further, women who experience perinatal IPV are also less likely to breastfeed and more likely to discontinue breastfeeding after 4 weeks of delivery.[31] The gravest risk is death of the fetus, baby, and mother. In a large national sample of women who had delivery-related discharges, women who reported perinatal IPV were 4 times more likely to have a stillbirth and 3 times more likely to have a delivery result in fetal death compared with nonabused peers.[32] Also, women exposed to IPV during pregnancy were 3 times more likely to be the victim of attempted or completed homicide compared with those who did not endorse perinatal IPV.[33] Clearly, the potential health outcomes associated with perinatal IPV are extensive and severe.

Perinatal IPV is associated with increased health care costs, utilization of emergency room visits during pregnancy, and receipt of care in the intensive care unit during pregnancy.[29] Unfortunately, women exposed to perinatal IPV are less likely to receive adequate prenatal care (ie, receive care after the fourth month of pregnancy or attended fewer than 50% of expected prenatal health care appointments).[34] Women exposed to IPV face several potential barriers to receiving medical treatment, including ongoing abuse, interpersonal and financial control from their perpetrator, economic stressors, and emotional barriers, such as shame.[35] It is essential to increase access to services among this population because IPV is often chronic and the negative consequences of perinatal IPV extend past the short-term impact on the infant to longer-term developmental issues.

LONG-TERM IMPACTS OF PERINATAL INTIMATE PARTNER VIOLENCE ON CHILDREN

Perinatal exposure to IPV has been shown to have long-term adverse consequences on children's mental, cognitive, and physical health. For instance, youth exposed to perinatal IPV are at an increased risk of developing subsequent internalizing and externalizing problems (eg, depression, anxiety, posttraumatic stress, low self-esteem, anger and irritability, risk-taking behaviors), and to struggle academically and socially.[36] Furthermore, health care utilization and costs for children with perinatal and postnatal exposure to IPV are higher and result in greater emergency department, primary care, and mental health visits.[37]

Executive Functioning

Pregnant women in abusive relationships are less likely to receive adequate prenatal care, have access to healthy foods, and are at increased risk of experiencing trauma-related stress, all of which has been linked to premature delivery, low birth weight, abnormal brain development, and impaired HPA axis functioning at birth and later in life.[38] As a result, perinatal exposure to IPV has been linked to long-term deficits in children's executive functioning (eg, impulsivity, poor decision making), cognitive functioning (eg, lower IQ levels and academic achievement), and delays in reaching appropriate neurodevelopmental milestones.[39] Exposure to IPV in the home from birth to age 3 years also has been associated with an increased risk of developing attention-deficit/hyperactivity disorder.[40] Thus, perinatal IPV can have lasting effects on multiple aspects of a child's executive functioning.

Attachment

Perinatal exposure to IPV also can have an adverse effect on mother-child interactions, or attachment. Perinatal IPV has been associated with less positive attunement to the infant, negative cognitions about parenting ability and self-efficacy, and decreased maternal responsiveness.[41] In turn, these can increase the risk of hostile interactions between the caregiver and child, and neglectful parenting practices.[42] It is important to understand the risks of perinatal IPV on the caregiver-child relationship, because relationships marked by qualities such as unpredictability, difficulty trusting, and unresponsiveness have been associated with increased risk of developing externalizing problems and risk-taking behaviors across the life span (eg, substance use, antisocial behavior, truancy).[43] Providing caregivers with histories of IPV resources related to parenting is essential to preventing difficulties in the caregiver-child relationship.

Exposure to Additional Adverse Events

Most individuals experience more than one potentially traumatic event across their lifetime, which is associated with more severe mental health symptoms.[11] Similarly, children exposed to IPV in the home are also at an increased risk of experiencing a wide range of adverse events, including physical abuse, sexual abuse, community violence, and bullying.[44] They also have a twofold increased risk of victimization or perpetration of IPV as adults. This demonstrates the cumulative impact that perinatal IPV may have on increasing risk for future exposure to adverse events across generations.

SUMMARY OF IMPACT

Perinatal IPV is associated with adverse mental health and obstetric health consequences for the mother, fetus, and child (**Table 1**). Although more research is needed to elucidate risk for the mental and obstetric health outcomes among pregnant women

Table 1	
Consequences that are associated with perinatal intimate partner violence	
Impact on mother's mental health	• Depression, posttraumatic stress disorder, anxiety • Substance use • Suicide
Impact on mother's obstetric health	• High blood pressure or edema • Vaginal bleeding • Severe nausea • Vomiting or dehydration • Kidney infection or urinary tract infection • Premature rupture of membranes • Placental abruption
Impact on mother and fetus/infant	• Miscarriage • Stillbirth • Fetal and mother death • Lower intrauterine growth and birth weight
Long-term impact on child	• Executive and cognitive functioning difficulties • Insecure and disorganized attachment • Exposure to additional traumatic events

according to timing and form of IPV, there is adequate support that violence experienced immediately before, during, and/or after pregnancy, as well as lifetime IPV, results in grave health consequences. Screening for IPV during perinatal care is essential to addressing the safety needs and obstetric health risks among this population.

PERINATAL INTIMATE PARTNER VIOLENCE SCREENING

The US Preventive Services Task Force recommends IPV screening for women of childbearing age, ensuring that such screening would have a moderate net public health benefit.[45] The Health Resources and Services Administration has developed guidelines into the Affordable Care Act that require routine IPV screening and counseling as a preventive service for adolescent and adult women.[46] Additional organizations, including the American Medical Association, American College of Obstetricians and Gynecologists, and the American Nurses Association have mandated screening for IPV across health care specialties. The Centers for Disease Control and Prevention outlines a list of all available screening tools for assessing IPV within health care settings (for a review of selected screening tools see **Table 2**).[47] There are several considerations to weigh when choosing a screening tool. Important considerations can include the following:

- Screening administration
- Type of IPV assessed
- Question types
- Cultural considerations

Screening Administration

Screening results can differ based on type of administration. Self-report measures can often increase the likelihood of disclosure and may remove potential administrator bias, which at times could sway patients to respond a particular way.[48] For example, if a provider has a full patient load that particular day, the provider may unintentionally send subtle messages to the patient to not endorse IPV (eg, no eye contact, reading

Table 2
Description of selected screening tools

Tool	Advantages	Disadvantages
Abuse Assessment Screen (AAS)	• 5 items assessing physical, sexual, and emotional abuse • Studied among pregnant women with good sensitivity (93%) • Spanish version available	• Specificity is low (55%) • Clinician administered only • Does not include behaviorally specific description of sexual violence
HITS	• 4 items with acronym to assist administration • Clinician or self-administered • Studied in family practice settings with good sensitivity (86%–96%) and specificity (91%–99%) • Spanish version available	• Limited to assessing physical intimate partner violence (IPV) and psychological IPV
STaT (slapped, things, and threaten)	• 3 items assessing physical violence and threats • Studied in emergency department with good sensitivity (96%) and specificity (75%)	• Limited to physical violence • Clinician administered only • Available for purchase
Ongoing violence assessment tool	• 4 items assessing physical and emotional IPV • Studied in emergency department with good sensitivity (86%–93%) and specificity (83%–86%)	• Self-report only • Focuses only on present abuse rather than lifetime

through screening questions quickly, asking questions as a negative). Provider-administered measures are also available, and potential benefits of provider-administered screening include building rapport and natural progression to safety planning. Therefore, it is important for each clinic to decide which administration of screening is preferred. There are many provider-administered screening tools that include standardized questions for providers to ask either all patients (universal screening) or patients who are at risk for IPV (targeted screening). Administration of screening when the partner is with the patient can further complicate the likelihood that an individual will report IPV; therefore, whenever possible, these screeners should be completed with the patient alone. This can be difficult to manage if a packet of screeners is provided to patients in the waiting room, as oftentimes perpetrators accompany their partners in the waiting room. Therefore, the timing and type of administration should be carefully considered for this sensitive topic.

Type of Intimate Partner Violence Assessed

When choosing a screening tool, it can be imperative to ensure that the types of IPV one is hoping to screen for are included in the measure. Not all measures of IPV include an assessment of physical, emotional, and sexual violence. Further, most screening questions do not assess for control of reproductive or sexual health. This may be important information to obtain after delivery when discussing future birth control methods. Therefore, individual clinics may decide to add questions to existing screeners.

Question Types

When assessing potentially traumatic events, like IPV, the questions used concerning violence exposure can be an important consideration. Screening tools rely on a series of questions that ask if someone has ever experienced a particular type of violence. Behaviorally specific questions that inquire if someone has ever had a particular experience (eg, "Has your partner ever strangled you?") can elicit more accurate responses than general questions (eg, "Has your partner ever abused you?"). Behaviorally specific questions have been informed by decades of research and generally yield more accurate responses.[47,48]

Cultural Considerations

There are important cultural considerations when choosing IPV screening tools. For example, in some cultures, there is a strong philosophy that IPV should be "kept in the family" and not discussed with those outside of the family. Therefore, it may be helpful to choose screeners that have been validated in ethnic minority populations. In addition, many screening tools assume that the individual is in a heteronormative monogamous relationship. Therefore, it may be important to assess what type of relationship(s) the individual is a part of before delivering the screening tool or to choose screening tools that do not assume the partner is male or that there is only one partner.

SAFETY PLANNING DURING PREGNANCY

If an individual receives a positive screen for IPV, safety planning can be an important next step. Depending on what the individual wants to do, safety planning may include safety within the relationship, safety while leaving the relationship, and safety after leaving the relationship. The following are some safety planning strategies that a provider can use to help the patient prepare for different situations based on the patient's willingness to leave the relationship.

If the individual is not willing to leave the relationship, safety planning may focus on *how to stay safe within the relationship*, which can include the following:

- Identifying safe areas of the home
- Gathering important documents, such as copies of birth certificates
- Making copies of important financial or ownership documents
- Providing assistance with contraceptive health and screening for sexual health issues
- Practicing how to escape if needed and to have an escape bag packed
- Identifying individuals to call in an emergency, including a local domestic violence shelter or national hotline with trained advocates, such as the Natural Disaster Violence Hotline

If the individual is preparing to leave the relationship, safety planning may focus on *how to safely leave the relationship*, which can include the following:

- Contacting a local domestic violence shelter or national hotline
- Documenting any injuries (provider can do this during the visit and place pictures in the medical record)
- Identifying a safe place to stay

If the individual has recently left the relationship, safety planning may focus on *how to stay safe after leaving the relationship*, which can include the following:

- Filing for a restraining order or order of protection
- Changing the route to work and/or school
- Changing the locks
- Alerting neighbors, family, coworkers, or school personnel to call the police if they see the perpetrator

The aforementioned screening tools can be used to assist with identifying when safety planning is needed.[47] After a positive screen or endorsement of IPV, safety planning checklists can be completed with the patient and provider. The National Coalition Against Domestic Violence (http://www.ncdsv.org/images/DV_Safety_Plan.pdf) provides a thorough safety planning checklist that includes several different strategies to assist in facilitating safety at various steps of responding to IPV.

REFERRAL TO TREATMENT

Evidence suggests that individuals are more likely to use interventions suggested by their health care provider[49] compared with any other official personnel. Additionally, pregnancy and preconceptional periods are times when women are most amenable to take advantage of interventions and make significant lifestyle changes. Importantly, findings have demonstrated that, at 2-year follow-up, women provided with referrals directly from the health care provider reported less violence and assault risk, as well as decreased health care costs.[50]

Depending on institution or clinic resources, intervention approaches can range from provider brief intervention and referral to treatment to "systems-level" approaches. A "systems-level" approach to intervention has proved most successful for IPV care.[51] Such approaches are designed to transform the entire organization to focus on IPV detection and care. The intervention areas of these programs aim to

1. Create a supportive environment
2. Link victims to community organizations
3. Provide systematic inquiry and referral integrated into the electronic health record
4. Provide on-site IPV services

However, not all clinics have the capability for on-site IPV services. Therefore, providers need to be well-informed regarding local resources, including local victim advocacy nonprofits, shelters, and national hotlines. Many local IPV organizations have information cards of local referrals that can be provided to patients. When offering referrals, providers should demonstrate patience and compassion, as it may take an individual exposed to IPV many visits before following up on recommendations. A "warm hand-off," where providers contact a local agency or national hotline on the phone with the patient in the office, can streamline connecting people to IPV referrals.

SUMMARY

IPV is a serious public health problem that involves various forms of physical and psychological aggression. Exposure to IPV has negative impacts on the body's stress response and autoimmune functioning, which may in part explain the association between perinatal IPV and a range of obstetric consequences, from increased vaginal bleeding to stillbirths. Although these health consequences typically come to the attention of providers, their relationship to IPV is much harder to detect. More research is needed to understand the mechanisms in which perinatal IPV leads to adverse obstetric outcomes. Given the ongoing nature of IPV, and the mental health sequelae, perinatal care is a critical period for providers to reach this population. Proper screening procedures, safety planning, and referrals are important methods to combat this public health problem.

REFERENCES

1. Breiding MJ, Basile KC, Smith SG, et al. Intimate partner violence surveillance: uniform definitions and recommended data elements, version 2.0. Atlanta

(GA): National Center for Injury Prevention and Control, Centers for Disease Control and Prevention; 2015.

2. Black MC, Basile KC, Breiding MJ, et al. The National Intimate Partner and Sexual Violence Survey (NISVS): 2010 summary report. Atlanta (GA): National Center for Injury Prevention and Control, Centers for Disease Control and Prevention; 2011.

3. Saltzman L, Johnson C, Gilbert B, et al. Physical abuse around the time of pregnancy: an examination of prevalence and risk factors in 16 states. Matern Child Health J 2003;7(1):31–43.

4. Silverman J, Decker M, Reed E, et al. Intimate partner violence victimization prior to and during pregnancy among women residing in 26 U.S. states: associations with maternal and neonatal health. Am J Obstet Gynecol 2006;195(1):140–8.

5. Bailey B, Daugherty R. Intimate partner violence during pregnancy: incidence and associated health behaviors in a rural population. Matern Child Health J 2007;11(5):495–503.

6. Flanagan J, Gordon K, Moore T, et al. Women's stress, depression, and relationship adjustment profiles as they relate to intimate partner violence and mental health during pregnancy and postpartum. Psychol Violence 2015;5(1):66–73.

7. Hellmuth J, Gordon K, Stuart G, et al. Women's intimate partner violence perpetration during pregnancy and postpartum. Matern Child Health J 2013;17(8): 1405–13.

8. Leone J, Lane S, Aubry R, et al. Effects of intimate partner violence on pregnancy trauma and placental abruption. J Womens Health (Larchmt) 2010;19(8):1501–9.

9. American Psychiatric Association. Diagnostic and statistical manual of mental disorders. 5th edition. Washington, DC: Author; 2013.

10. Hedtke K, Ruggiero K, Kilpatrick D, et al. A longitudinal investigation of interpersonal violence in relation to mental health and substance use. J Consult Clin Psychol 2008;76(4):633–47. Available at: MEDLINE. Ipswich (MA).

11. Kilpatrick D, Resnick H, Milanak M, et al. National estimates of exposure to traumatic events and PTSD prevalence using DSM-IV and DSM-5 criteria. J Trauma Stress 2013;26(5):537–47.

12. Dutton M, Green B, Kaltman S, et al. Intimate partner violence, PTSD, and adverse health outcomes. J Interpers Violence 2006;21(7):955–68.

13. Kastello J, Jacobsen K, Gaffney K, et al. Posttraumatic stress disorder among low-income women exposed to perinatal intimate partner violence: posttraumatic stress disorder among women exposed to partner violence. Arch Womens Ment Health 2016;19(3):521–8.

14. Connelly C, Hazen A, Baker-Ericzén M, et al. Is screening for depression in the perinatal period enough? The co-occurrence of depression, substance abuse, and intimate partner violence in culturally diverse pregnant women. J Womens Health (Larchmt) 2013;22(10):844–52.

15. Beydoun H, Al-Sahab B, Beydoun M, et al. Intimate partner violence as a risk factor for postpartum depression among Canadian women in the Maternity Experience Survey. Ann Epidemiol 2010;20(8):575–83.

16. Melville JL, Gavin A, Guo Y, et al. Depressive disorders during pregnancy: prevalence and risk factors in a large urban sample. Obstet Gynecol 2010;116(5): 1064–70.

17. Cerulli C, Talbot N, Tang W, et al. Co-occurring intimate partner violence and mental health diagnoses in perinatal women. J Womens Health (Larchmt) 2011; 20(12):1797–803.

18. Gelaye B, Kajeepeta S, Williams M. Suicidal ideation in pregnancy: an epidemiologic review. Arch Womens Ment Health 2016;19(5):741–51.

19. Tabb K, Huang H, Faisal-Cury A, et al. Intimate partner violence is associated with suicidality among low-income postpartum women. J Womens Health (Larchmt) 2017;24:2017.

20. Palladino CL, Singh V, Campbell J, et al. Homicide and suicide during the perinatal period: findings from the national violent death reporting system. Obstet Gynecol 2011;118(5):1056–63.

21. Scribano P, Stevens J, Kaizar E. The effects of intimate partner violence before, during, and after pregnancy in nurse visited first time mothers. Matern Child Health J 2013;17(2):307–18.

22. Martin S, Beaumont J, Kupper L. Substance use before and during pregnancy: links to intimate partner violence. Am J Drug Alcohol Abuse 2003;29(3):599–617.

23. Khantzian EJ. The self-medication hypothesis of substance use disorders: reconsideration and recent applications. Harv Rev Psychiatry 1997;4:231–44.

24. Sullivan T, Holt L. PTSD symptom clusters are differentially related to substance use among community women exposed to intimate partner violence. J Trauma Stress 2008;21(2):173–80.

25. Cheng D, Salimi S, Terplan M, et al. Intimate partner violence and maternal cigarette smoking before and during pregnancy. Obstet Gynecol 2015;125(2):356–62 (smoking cig 24).

26. Rodriguez M, Heilemann M, Fielder E, et al. Intimate partner violence, depression, and PTSD among pregnant Latina women. Ann Fam Med 2008;6(1):44–52.

27. Flynn H, Walton M, Chermack S, et al. Brief detection and co-occurrence of violence, depression and alcohol risk in prenatal care settings. Arch Womens Ment Health 2007;10(4):155–61.

28. Agrawal A, Ickovics J, Lewis J, et al. Postpartum intimate partner violence and health risks among young mothers in the United States: a prospective study. Matern Child Health J 2014;18(8):1985–92.

29. Mogos M, Araya W, Masho S, et al. The feto-maternal health cost of intimate partner violence among delivery-related discharges in the United States, 2002-2009. J Interpers Violence 2016;31(3):444–64.

30. Yost N, Bloom S, McIntire D, et al. A prospective observational study of domestic violence during pregnancy. Obstet Gynecol 2005;106(1):61–5.

31. Silverman JG, Decker MR, Reed E, et al. Intimate partner violence around the time of pregnancy: association with breastfeeding behavior. J Womens Health (Larchmt) 2006;15(8):934–40.

32. Murphy C, Schei B, Myhr T, et al. Abuse: a risk factor for low birth weight? A systematic review and meta-analysis. CMAJ 2001;164(11):1567–72.

33. McFarlane J, Campbell J, Sharps P, et al. Abuse during pregnancy and femicide: urgent implications for women's health. Obstet Gynecol 2002;100(1):27–36.

34. Cha S, Masho S. Intimate partner violence and utilization of prenatal care in the United States. J Interpers Violence 2014;29(5):911–27.

35. Rodríguez M, Valentine J, Son J, et al. Intimate partner violence and barriers to mental health care for ethnically diverse populations of women. Trauma Violence Abuse 2009;10(4):358–74.

36. Carlson B. Children exposed to intimate partner violence: research findings and implications for intervention. Trauma Violence Abuse 2000;1(4):321–42.

37. Rivara F, Anderson M, Thompson R, et al. Intimate partner violence and health care costs and utilization for children living in the home. Pediatrics 2007;120(6):1270–7.

38. Entringer S, Kumsta R, Hellhammer D, et al. Prenatal exposure to maternal psychosocial stress and HPA axis regulation in young adults. Horm Behav 2009; 55(2):292–8.

39. Aarnoudse-Moens C, Weisglas-Kuperus N, van Goudoever J, et al. Meta-analysis of neurobehavioral outcomes in very preterm and/or very low birth weight children. Pediatrics 2009;124(2):717–28.

40. Bauer N, Gilbert A, Carroll A, et al. Associations of early exposure to intimate partner violence and parental depression with subsequent mental health outcomes. JAMA Pediatr 2013;167(4):341–7.

41. Huth-Bocks AC, Krause K, Ahlfs-Dunn S, et al. Relational trauma and posttraumatic stress symptoms among pregnant women. Psychodyn Psychiatry 2013; 41:277–301.

42. Cox S, Hopkins J, Hans S. Attachment in preterm infants and their mothers: neonatal risk status and maternal representations. Infant Ment Health J 2000; 21(6):464–80. Available at: PsycINFO. Ipswich (MA).

43. Fearon R, Bakermans-Kranenburg M, van IJzendoorn M, et al. The significance of insecure attachment and disorganization in the development of children's externalizing behavior: a meta-analytic study. Child Dev 2010;81(2):435–56.

44. Holt S, Buckley H, Whelan S. The impact of exposure to domestic violence on children and young people: a review of the literature. Child Abuse Negl 2008; 32(8):797–810.

45. Moyer VA, US Preventive Services Task Force. Screening for intimate partner violence and abuse of elderly and vulnerable adults: U.S. Preventive Services Task Force recommendation statement. Ann Intern Med 2013;158(6):478–86. Rockville (MD).

46. Oehme K, Stern N. Case for mandatory training on screening for domestic violence in the wake of the Affordable Care Act. The. U. Pa. JL & Soc. Change 2014;17(1). Available at: https://www.google.com/url?sa=t&rct=j&q=&esrc=s& source=web&cd=1&cad=rja&uact=8&ved=0ahUKEwiP0eWxhf7aAhVDhOAKHZ FEC7oQFggsMAA&url=https%3A%2F%2Fscholarship.law.upenn.edu%2Fcgi% 2Fviewcontent.cgi%3Farticle%3D1162%26context%3Djlasc&usg=AOvVaw2j3n4 o2okqWWyoslzWHy3Y. Accessed May 11, 2018.

47. Basile KC, Hertz MF, Back SE. Intimate partner violence and sexual violence victimization assessment instruments for use in healthcare settings: version 1. Atlanta (GA): Centers for Disease Control and Prevention, National Center for Injury Prevention and Control; 2007.

48. National Research Council. Potential sources of error: Nonresponse, specification, and measurement. Estimating the incidence of rape and sexual assault. In: Kruttschnitt C, Kalsbeek WD, House CC, editors. Panel on measuring rape and sexual assault in Bureau of Justice household surveys. Washington, DC: The National Academies Press; 2014. p. 127–38.

49. McCloskey L, Lichter E, Williams C, et al. Assessing intimate partner violence in health care settings leads to women's receipt of interventions and improved health. Public Health Rep 2006;121(4):435–44.

50. McFarlane J, Groff J, O'Brien J, et al. Secondary prevention of intimate partner violence: a randomized controlled trial. Nurs Res 2006;55(1):52–61.

51. Miller E, McCaw B, Humphreys B, et al. Integrating intimate partner violence assessment and intervention into healthcare in the United States: a systems approach. J Womens Health (Larchmt) 2015;24(1):92–9.

The Unwelcome Guest
Working with Childhood Sexual Abuse Survivors in Reproductive Health Care

Phyllis M. Florian, PsyD

KEYWORDS

- Childhood sexual abuse • Reproductive health care • Trauma • Providers

KEY POINTS

- Health care providers (HCPs), in service of best care practices, are often poorly prepared to respond to childhood sexual abuse (CSA) survivors' specific needs in reproductive health care.
- With few legitimized protocols addressing the CSA survivor population, HCPs struggle with delivering appropriate interventions that meet professional standards of care within the systemic constraints of reproductive health care.
- To bridge the gap that exists when the unwelcome guest of CSA enters the reproductive health care arena, it is important to understand the psychological influences of trauma that affect CSA survivors, the symptoms or behavioral cues that are commonly revealed, and therapeutic approaches that can facilitate positive patient-provider experiences in health care.

Health care providers (HCPs) undergo rigorous training in service of clinical competency excellence in all specialties of practice. In women's reproductive health care, this clinical competency demands attentiveness to multiple organic systems and complex factors affecting the overall well-being of women, especially expectant mothers and their babies. Reproductive HCPs—that is, obstetricians/gynecologists, midwives, and labor and delivery nurses—engage patients in a joint mission to encourage wellness in all aspects of reproductive health care.

When patients have histories of adverse childhood events (ie, neglect, verbal, physical, or sexual abuse, as described in the Adverse Childhood Experiences Study: https://www.cdc.gov/violenceprevention/acestudy/index.html), their lived experiences of initiating and using reproductive health care may be tenuous. Some women with histories of adverse childhood events are less inclined to access routine or preventive health care.[1] Even with sufficient health insurance, they may prefer to avoid the

Disclosure Statement: The author has no commercial or financial conflicts of interest and identifies no special funding sources outside of her private practice income.
Prospicare, 555 West Crosstown Parkway, Suite 403, Kalamazoo, MI 49008, USA
E-mail address: dr.phyllisflorian@prospicare.com

Obstet Gynecol Clin N Am 45 (2018) 549–562
https://doi.org/10.1016/j.ogc.2018.04.009
0889-8545/18/© 2018 Elsevier Inc. All rights reserved.

clinical setting altogether.[1] Others seek out medical services for largely unexplained physical symptoms, giving significant attention to somatic complaints and demanding answers from HCPs.[2] These patients may be hypervigilant and sensitive toward all aspects of their bodies.[3] Conversely, patients may be reluctant to adhere to prescribed health care practices—particularly if they are depressed or perceive themselves to be helpless or unworthy.[4] These scenarios are especially true for survivors of childhood sexual abuse (CSA). From the standpoint of both HCPs and patients, CSA is a significant factor that complicates the mission of wellness in reproductive health care. Most often, these factors complicate the provider-patient relationship and are heightened by gaps in communication, expectations, and unmet needs for both parties.

The incidence and qualitative experience of CSA survivors in reproductive health care settings have been studied, primarily in the past 2 decades. Recent statistics suggest that CSA history is as common in reproductive health care settings as gestational diabetes and hypertension.[5] Concurrently, a movement toward trauma-informed health care has been launched in social service agencies, clinical settings, and educational programs. Trauma-informed protocol is supplemental or adjunct training to standard clinical skills. It is fitting to explore the current experience of reproductive HCPs vis-à-vis CSA survivors who become their patients and to offer trauma-informed recommendations for better provider-patient experiences.

EMOTIONAL OVERVIEW OF THE CHILDHOOD SEXUAL ABUSE SURVIVOR

Reproductive HCPs conduct their professional trade in the physical proximity of body parts that are intimately tied to multiple layers of meaning for most women. Breasts and genitalia are sensual and sensitive as well as utilitarian—for sexual pleasure, for birthing and nourishing babies, and for supporting the health of the next generation. Reproductive HCPs work daily with these body parts, having acquired a biological mastery of, and a learned familiarity with, breasts and internal and external reproductive organs. Conversely, CSA survivors regard their body parts with a different level of meaning: violation, trauma, and horrific memories, and this is where they push back from most attempts to befriend or become personally comfortable with these physical body parts; there will always be that dark cloud that hangs over their perceptions of breasts and genitalia.

It is specifically because of how these women carry the memories of CSA into adulthood that their bodies are often the containers of mixed messages, emotional ambivalence, painful secrets, and multiple layers of meaning. The physical body may even feel like the enemy that CSA survivors must reconcile on a daily basis to manage physically being in the world.

FROM THE PERSPECTIVE OF THE CHILDHOOD SEXUAL ABUSE SURVIVOR

Research from the National Child Traumatic Stress Network suggests that 1 of 4 girls and 1 of 6 boys experience sexual abuse in one form or another before the age of 18 (http://nctsn.org/nctsn_assets/pdfs/caring/ChildSexualAbuseFactSheet.pdf). Because CSA is often held in secrecy, however, many cases are never reported. CSA is disturbing by its nature and traumatic for its victims. Many CSA survivors reach adulthood without revealing the stories of their abuse.

Survivors often relegate memories of such unsettling childhood events to past history in an effort to protect themselves from the burden of re-experiencing painful and sometimes unclear or confusing memories. Studies indicate that women who access reproductive health care may avoid or omit disclosure of CSA during the intake process and, in many cases, during routine obstetrics and gynecology (OB/GYN) health screenings.[3,6,7] In adulthood, many CSA survivors are more than happy to detach from the memories of abuse during formative years. "That was then; this is now" is a rationale that allows survivors to compartmentalize past experiences while protecting their current psychological vulnerabilities.[8–10] Some survivors truly believe that, as fully-fledged adults, they have no need to report information about experiences that occurred many years ago. Ironically, this secrecy sometimes parallels or affirms the directives they were given by their perpetrators, years ago: "Don't tell anybody!" It was a mandate for safety back then, and CSA survivors may continue to affirm it in adulthood. Not telling is often a mechanism for self-protection.

Additionally, HCPs may find themselves surprised by the intensity of patient reactions during clinical procedures that seem routine and minimally invasive. CSA survivor-patients may be reacting to subconscious triggers and have no conscious awareness of their own history of CSA, due to suppressed memories from horrific childhood events.[8,11] It is important to acknowledge that some CSA survivors may stifle memories about their own abuse. These memories are often buried in the recesses of the mind, where specific details are unclear and even inaccessible.[12] CSA survivors may engage in active "not wanting to know"[13] because they are not psychologically prepared to address the implications of fully recognizing their trauma histories. When CSA occurs during very early childhood (especially during preverbal development), patients may have no conscious recollections of abuse.

FACTORS AFFECTING CHILDHOOD SEXUAL ABUSE SURVIVORS IN REPRODUCTIVE HEALTH CARE

- CSA survivors may verbally admit or demonstrate extreme reluctance to be physically touched or examined by an HCP.
- CSA survivors may feel ashamed of their bodies because of unresolved psychological distress brought on by childhood abuse.
- CSA survivors may fear the pain of pelvic examinations, labor, and/or childbirth as mimicking the pain endured through childhood abuse.
- CSA survivors may hope to breastfeed their babies but are more likely to abandon this option earlier than those mothers not affected by CSA—likely due to the psychological distress related to mixed messages about their own breasts and the sensations of breastfeeding.[9,14]

Table 1	
Observable behaviors characteristic of unresolved childhood sexual abuse and related trauma	
Observable Behavior	**Characteristics**
Hyperarousal	• Sleeping problems, not associated with a newborn in the home • Difficulty concentrating • Irritability and/or angry outbursts • Anxiety or panic episodes, especially in response to or in anticipation of invasive procedures
Hypervigilance	• Sensitivity to a perceived threat, as if on high alert • Guardedness • Heightened awareness of surroundings and people; may be manifest in tracking secondary providers/personnel in the clinical office or delivery room • Sensory sensitivity to touch—via provider's hands or clinical instruments
	(continued on next page)

Table 1 (continued)	
Observable Behavior	**Characteristics**
Hyperreactivity	• Exaggerated startle response • Over-the-top response to sensory stimuli—most often in the clinical setting, during any touch • Jumpiness when someone enters the room, when instruments make noises, and so forth
Avoidance	• Refusing to report or discuss CSA history • Shying away from routine clinical procedures • Not making eye contact with the provider; reluctant to wear gown or use stirrups • Not following through with prescribed aftercare, medications, or follow-up visits
Amnesia	• Literally unable to recall something that happened in the past; may occur in CSA, especially when it occurred in very early childhood
Anhedonia	• Reduced ability to experience pleasure • Social withdrawal, or lack of social relationships—may be at risk for poor support in postpartum care • Negative feelings toward self and others • Loss of libido or interest in physical intimacy, may report decrease in sexual interest or frequency of relations, increased marital problems • Persistent physical problems—somatic complaints that require clinical attention
Psychic numbing	• A psychological defense mechanism • Occurs when the conscious experience is so overwhelming and/or emotionally painful that the person shuts off and becomes numb • Often occurs when gynecologic procedures mimic past CSA/trauma • May be likened to a psychological anesthesia • Loss of emotions as social signals/loss of stimulus discrimination—a critical concern during postpartum care of newborns, for example, • Inability to engage in meaningful, collaborative dialogue during physical examination
Dissociation	• A defense mechanism to escape identification with the current circumstance—CSA survivors may acknowledge feeling as if they had left the room during certain procedures • Providers perceive patients to be checked out when this occurs, usually as a result of procedures that retraumatize a CSA survivor—no eye contact, no dialog, unable to participate in collaborative health care decisions in a dissociative state
Depersonalization	• Patient experiences herself as an observer of her body in the room • Feeling robotic, not in control of what is going on; merely an observer
Derealization	• Patient feels alienated or disconnected from surroundings, as if watching a movie • Emotionally disconnected; like being separated by a glass wall
Traumatic re-experiencing	• Flooding of CSA memories, usually triggered by a sensory experience that is similar in perceived danger—for example, pelvic examination, birthing experience, breast examination • Flashbacks—quite disturbing to the CSA survivor • Patient is psychologically back in the place of the original trauma, behaves as if the trauma is rehappening or being repeated; increased emotional responses, physical guardedness, panic or terror response

FROM THE PERSPECTIVE OF THE REPRODUCTIVE HEALTH CARE PROVIDER

In reproductive health care, this "not telling/not knowing" puts HCPs at a distinct disadvantage, especially when routine gynecologic procedures quickly evolve into highly emotional, antagonistic, or disengaging experiences with patients. Providers are often caught unaware, scrambling to negotiate variables that complicate standard procedures. They are forced to juggle, on the one hand, their philosophic commitment to professional standards and compassion in all aspects of patient care and, on the other hand, pressing issues of time management, clinical/psychosocial resources for the patient, and so forth—all the while engaging in the exact gynecologic procedures that trigger these specific patients. In a split second, business as usual may become crisis management. Is it any wonder that reproductive HCPs, when unaware of the specific psychosocial factors of CSA survivorship, may assess these patients as difficult to work with or intentionally noncompliant?

In some cases, the first indication or suspicion of a patient's CSA history might occur when a routine gynecologic examination is performed, and a patient's reactions seem inconsistent with the purpose of the examination and the relative discomfort of the procedure for most OB/GYN patients.

Behaviors that may lead to a suspicion of patients having a CSA history may include difficulty dropping their knees so that the pelvic examination can be completed or becoming tearful, angry, or dissociative during routine gynecologic procedures. Such suspicions can be transferred to partners who are in the room with the patients, wondering if these partners might be contributing to the suspected abuse. These sorts of behaviors may be cues to a history of CSA despite patients denying this factor in their self-reported history.

HCPs anticipate—and may expect—that most patients are forthcoming with information that may affect the course of their reproductive health care. Unfortunately, that is not often the reality with CSA survivors. This secrecy can create frustration, uncertainty, and, sometimes, even anger on the part of the HCP.

Ironically, some patients believe that their reproductive HCPs have great professional acuity; they expect the providers to be able to see that they are CSA survivors without verbally reporting or affirming this information. The expectations from patients are grounded in the perception of providers as all-knowing trained professionals. They expect providers to get it and then repair any misunderstandings in the clinical setting.[15]

HCPs often wrestle with the decision to say anything to their patients whom they suspect to have a CSA history. Some decide to engage their patients in a dialog about the suspected CSA, whereas others do not wish to initiate the conversation at all. Providers weigh their options about investigating CSA history based on many variables (eg, time/time management and practice schedules, patient relations, and familiarity or comfort with the subject matter) that inform their initial response. These variables come to the forefront when HCPs initially determine their own sense of urgency to know about suspected CSA history. The desire to compassionately get information about possible CSA can create significant pressures in the busy clinical setting. Furthermore, HCPs may have concerns about their clinical scope of professional training in directly verbalizing their suspicions of CSA or in responding effectively to a patient's affirmative revelation of CSA. It is easy to assume that if a patient is not saying anything, she is not being her own advocate, and then it is not the HCPs responsibility to bring it up—especially in situations where the HCP is keenly aware that another patient is waiting. Refraining from investigating CSA suspicions seems to be in service of HCPs trying to protect themselves from diving into patient issues beyond the scope of traditional reproductive health care, beyond intervention strategies that HCPs are trained to provide in reproductive health care settings.

Reproductive HCPs have identified specific themes from their experiences of working with CSA survivor-patients (discussed later).

The Process of Knowing

HCPs experience this coming to an awareness through a dynamic process: first, through observations of a patient's behavioral and emotional cues and then to internally questioning these cues and drawing on lived experiences as a professional in reproductive health care, toward intuitively knowing that a patient is a survivor. This process occurs in a short period of real time. Some HCPs describe this as professional intuition about CSA patients, and it is a learned skill.

External Pressures

External pressures are factors that influence a provider's decision making. The 2 pressures include time pressures (ie, scheduling policies and procedures that restrict the amount of time providers may give each patient and the time pressure to act immediately on patient distress) and systems pressures (ie, managed health care scheduling practices, conversion to electronic medical records, hierarchy rankings, standards of care, continuous quality improvement while avoiding liability issues, and so forth) that demand accountability in all decisions.

Powerlessness/Helplessness

A CSA survivor's presentation in the clinical setting challenges the sense of mastery and competence that HCPs require to do their work effectively. They feel powerless to slow down time in service of navigating this phenomenon in a manner that gives respect to the level of CSA survivorship that each patient may experience. In some cases, HCPs express deep concern that their actions may be hurting or, worse, retraumatizing CSA survivors. HCPs acknowledge that they are not equipped to treat many emotional and psychosocial problems that may emerge in their clinical setting—particularly regarding such traumatic historical events. This powerless/helpless feeling does not diminish HCPs' empathy for the CSA survivor-patients in their care.

Ambivalent Emotions

HCPs express sympathy, pity, and/or empathy for the patients who are CSA survivors. They acknowledge anger that CSA exists as a social reality at all. Concurrently, HCPs experience frustration for the provider-patient process, especially when these difficult patients do not know or say what they need—leaving providers keenly aware of the failure of communication with their patients and searching for options that confirm their expertise in the reproductive arena and in their work with CSA survivor situations. They also affirm their desire to help these patients, while contending with professional demands of interpersonal boundaries, time constraints in managed care settings, and personal integrity.

Action Plan Through Adaptations

HCPs create plans of action by making adaptations in protocol and individualizing the experience for the sake of each CSA survivor-patient. This action plan through adaptation is often completed in split-second decision-making. Whether they explicitly engage in acknowledgment of the CSA history or simply adjust their methodology in accomplishing the procedures of reproductive health, the providers intentionally change their approach to each CSA survivor in service of a more collaborative provider-patient dyad.[16]

To bridge the gap that exists when the unwelcome guest of CSA enters the reproductive health care arena, it is important to understand the psychological influences of trauma that affect CSA survivors, the symptoms or behavioral cues that are commonly revealed, and the lived experiences of the HCPs that serve these women.

SYMPTOMS OF CHILDHOOD SEXUAL ABUSE MANIFEST IN REPRODUCTIVE HEALTH CARE

In the reproductive health care arena, multiple observable behaviors are characteristic of unresolved CSA and related trauma. The list presented in **Table 1** is not exhaustive.[2,3,17-20]

Given the breadth of symptoms that may be presented in the reproductive health care setting, it behooves HCPs not only to be familiar with these indicators but also to become comfortable in acknowledging and addressing them.

THE HEALTH CARE PROVIDER'S EXPERIENCE

Research has shown that HCPs often experience mixed emotions when confronting this unwelcome guest in their arena of expertise. Many HCPs consider dealing with CSA survivors emotionally, physically, and psychologically taxing.[16] This may lead to vicarious traumatization—a process by which the caregiver may experience trauma personally, by emotional and/or physical proximity to the traumatized person or event. For trauma-service personnel—firefighters, police officers, and emergency room medical staff—this experience is an accepted, daily aspect of trauma stewardship—defined as "a daily practice through which individuals...tend to the hardship, pain, or trauma experienced by humans."[21] Reproductive HCPs face varying levels of trauma stewardship and are prone to vicarious trauma because of their exposure to complications and particularly dramatic or stressful events in the workplace. This vicarious traumatization is exacerbated by certain psychosocial factors, which may affect HCPs. Invariably, some HCPs are CSA survivors themselves. Others know somebody who has been personally affected by sexual abuse or assault.[16] Ongoing exposure to this difficult phenomenon has the potential to further complicate interactions with patients who show symptoms of unresolved CSA. It is imperative for HCPs to recognize their own vicarious trauma symptoms, and to seek help for symptoms that they cannot manage independently.[21]

SIGNS OF VICARIOUS TRAUMATIZATION IN HEALTH CARE PROVIDERS

This list is neither exhaustive nor exclusive to reproductive HCPs (**Table 2**). It behooves all HCPs to recognize when the stresses related to roles as providers of care negatively affect the quality of that care or the quality of their lives.

WHAT CAN HEALTH CARE PROVIDERS DO TO IMPROVE CARE OF CHILDHOOD SEXUAL ABUSE PATIENTS?

Parallel processes occur between CSA survivors and those caregivers who may be vulnerable to vicarious traumatization. In both cases, individuals need to assert the desire to be validated and respected, affirm a sense of control for themselves, and establish intentional engagement in the moment. For both parties, this is the

Table 2
Signs of vicarious traumatization in health care providers

Symptoms of Vicarious Traumatization	Situational Settings/Description
• Anxiety or panic attacks	• Occurring prior to work or during the work day, with specific patients
• Hypervigilance; fear of what might be there	• Looking for anything unusual in patient presentations, and what it might mean regarding CSA history
• Diminished creativity in patient care	• Diminished ability to be innovative or flexible in procedures or protocols with patients
• Diminished ability to handle complications; OR • Hero complex	• Shutting down when complications occur OR • The need to be the one who rescues or saves the suffering patient (at all cost to HCP self-care)

• Social isolation during personal time
  OR
• Over-volunteerism and over-engagement
	• Decreased desire to be around loved ones, friends
	  OR
	• Making oneself available for volunteer opportunities, constantly offering to help/fix/resolve when it is not required; not knowing how to say "no"

• Moments of dissociation	• Checking out mentally, particularly after being triggered by something emotionally intolerable in the moment • Working on autopilot without authentically engaging with the patient; going through the motions
• Minimizing or discounting another's experience	• Described as a "suck it up, Buttercup" response; growing intolerance for patients' complaints
• Numbing	• No longer feeling happy or sad; diminished ability to empathize with patients
• Anger	• Cynicism toward work, patients, even loved ones at home
• Avoidance	• Losing interest in actively listening or engaging with the patient; avoiding complex conversations; ignoring one's own feelings
• Extreme fatigue	• Physical exhaustion that does not respond to a good night's sleep
• Engaging in addictive behaviors	Drinking, smoking, drugging, overeating, accessing porn—any behaviors that are disordered, used to avoid feelings related to trauma, or perceived failure in professional roles

foundation of effective provider-patient interactions. Acknowledging that "we are all in this together" is a helpful first step.

FEELING SAFE THROUGH VALIDATION AND RESPECT

CSA survivors who access reproductive health care feel especially vulnerable and worry about how OB/GYN procedures might trigger memories. The need to feel safe is important to all survivors of trauma[17]; in the clinical setting, it is paramount for CSA survivors. How do HCPs establish this sense of safety for patients?

First, HCPs should presume that any patient may have a CSA history. They can approach patient interactions with words and behavior that convey an interest in the individuality of each patient, developing rapport. Often, this creates a safe space for CSA survivors to share their concerns or histories. HCPs, while affirming their professional competencies, are more effective when they convey present-focused awareness and openness to a patient's perspective. Above all, HCPs convey safety to CSA survivors when they communicate the limitations of their own training (ie, they are NOT experts in behavioral health or trauma treatment), while affirming a desire to help each CSA survivor find professional support as needed, through referrals, consultations, and other interventions.

Women in labor and delivery, in particular, need to gain control to assert self-determination during this most intimate experience. Control is an important coping strategy, particularly for dealing with invasive procedures. The loss of control potentially causes more distress than the procedure itself.[22]

Women who are CSA survivors may find it especially difficult to trust their caregivers, yet a good relationship between the HCP and CSA survivor is critically important to successfully navigate their reproductive health care. To establish that trust, it is necessary for HCPs to have open communication; it requires validation of the CSA survivors' experiences, recognition of distress, and a need to listen for the frequently unspoken messages.[23]

CSA survivors feel safer and more at ease with HCPs who convey a willingness to slow down the process of many health care procedures, particularly during labor and delivery. Other beneficial aspects of the interpersonal affiliation that HCPs may have with CSA survivors include accomplishing goals with intentionality, accessibility, collaborative dialog, and, most importantly, respect for the patient's vulnerabilities. Respecting the patient this way, HCPs affirm the agency each CSA survivor can have in taking charge of her own wellness.

TRAUMA-INFORMED HEALTH CARE: AN OVERVIEW

Health care systems that are trauma-informed acknowledge the pervasive, often insidious, influence of CSA history (as well as other childhood traumas) on the process of healthcare practices with adults. Trauma-informed health care systems proactively integrate knowledge about trauma into their policies and procedures, staff trainings, and clinical practices. The goal of trauma-informed health care is to raise awareness among all HCPs and support staff who interact with patients, that many patients may have some form of trauma history; better outcomes are possible when providers and staff presume the need for a trauma-informed approach to each patient. The Substance Abuse and Mental Health Services Administration of the United States government (www.samhsa.gov) has put forth 6 key principles of trauma-informed health care. These include a conveyance of safety; trustworthy practices and transparency in service delivery; collaboration between provider and patient; peer support; empowerment; and cultural, historical, and gender sensitivity for all patients and related participants in clinical settings (https://www.samhsa. gov/nctic/trauma-interventions).

Trauma-informed treatment interventions for CSA survivors also include awareness of frequently co-occurring disorders, such as substance abuse, mood disorders, sexual health problems, body-image problems, and interpersonal/primary relationship problems. Many of these disorders are the result of long-term maladaptive coping strategies, first implemented in childhood to survive traumatic events. These coping strategies became survival tools during childhood events and are now tenaciously — although often subconsciously—held in adulthood. Sensitive, collaborative care for CSA survivors includes attention to individual styles of coping, engagement of spouses/partners as patient allies (unless contraindicated because of partner abuse), and use of multiple resources for overall patient well-being.

TRAUMA-INFORMED REPRODUCTIVE HEALTH CARE: SUGGESTIONS FOR BEST PRACTICES

- Although the HCP is the expert in reproductive health care, the patient is the best expert of herself. When the HCP shifts the power dynamics (as the patient may be perceiving them), to convey a desire to learn from the patient's expertise, the HCP invites her into a collaborative process, in service of best care practices. This perceived power shift also permits the CSA survivor to gain a sense of trust and to be forthcoming with information, empowering the patient over time.
- The HCP respectfully verbalizes what is noticed from the patient's actions, emotions, and behavioral cues, asking early, asking gently, and asking again throughout the relationship with this patient, because the HCP may be emotionally shut out until the patient develops a sense of trust.
- The HCP is challenged to consider modifications to procedures and interventions, when situations demand this. If a patient's distress or resistance is noticed, the HCP should be willing to change the pace of what is being done, conveying respect and a desire for a collaborative process. If possible, the HCP offers to stop the procedure and come back to it at a later time, encouraging appropriate self-care measures to re-establish her sense of personal comfort and safety:
    - You look a little distressed. How can I help you through this procedure?
    - Can you tell me how you are doing? You seem to be protecting yourself, and I want to respect your needs.
    - I can tell this is difficult for you. Would you like me to pause or stop for a few minutes? Would you like to reschedule this procedure (if possible)?
- The HCP establishes a collaborative plan/protocol for the CSA survivor-patient's triggering situations/sensations. What are her triggers? When she is triggered, what does she need in this setting to take care of herself? Are there any procedures, positions, or interventions that are strictly unacceptable for her? Does she have a phrase or word that will signal the HCP to pause what is being done? Has she defined a safe place (real or imagined) that she can mentally access, if a necessary procedure or process is triggering or frightening for her?
- The HCP articulates with empathy that the HCP is sorry the patient has suffered in the past, telling the patient that her history of CSA is beyond the scope of the HCP's expertise. Honesty matters most, especially if the HCP conveys willingness to find experts, knowing which resources can support the patient, and affirming that the patient is not being passed off (**Table 3**). The HCP follows-up with this patient to confirm that she has found the resources that work for her, congratulating her on taking steps to regain control of her life this way.

- The HCP practices techniques of mindfulness interventions: breathing with patients, maintaining eye contact, and modeling the intentional presence the HCP wants the patient to use. The HCP uses breathing patterns associated with labor and delivery coaching—even for nonpregnant patients. The HCP stays on the same physical level as the patient whenever possible, to affirm provider-patient attunement. When modeling mindfulness techniques for patients, HCPs may concurrently help themselves mitigate their situational stressors.
- The HCP provides compassionate authority as needed, with validation of patient distress/discomfort and empathy for what the patient is feeling in the moment. As needed, the HCP provides rational, sound reasons for continuing certain invasive procedures and why/how they can be successfully accomplished.

Table 3
Examples of resources for survivors of childhood sexual abuse and related trauma

Patient Issue or Need	Referral Options
Mood disorder—depression or anxiety—and/or history of mental health condition	Therapist (psychologist or licensed clinical social worker) who specializes in perinatal mood disorders—Postpartum Support International has state and regional representatives and provider directories
CSA history	Trauma-informed mental health provider—private practice listings (eg, through provider networks: https://www.psychologytoday.com/us/therapists?tr=Hdr_SubBrand)
Socioeconomic stress—housing, employment, and so forth	Community-based social service agencies, nonprofit housing advocacy groups, social service case managers
Domestic violence	YWCA domestic assault programs, safe shelters
Sexual assault (recent)	Rape crisis center
Other needs	Medical social worker

- The HCP provides advocacy for CSA survivor-patients: making referrals to in-house medical social workers, trauma-informed therapists, case managers, and so forth. When partners or other family members are present, the HCP affirms the CSA survivor-patient as the primary focus, conveying utmost respect for patient.

MOVING FORWARD

Women with CSA history may be transformed by positive provider-patient experiences of trauma-informed, effective reproductive health care. Educational systems that generate competent providers in reproductive health must acknowledge and wholeheartedly endorse trauma-informed training in CSA and posttraumatic stress disorder.

TOP 10 RECOMMENDATIONS FOR TREATING CHILDHOOD SEXUAL ABUSE SURVIVORS IN REPRODUCTIVE HEALTH CARE

The following recommendations are intended to encourage changes in how CSA are treated in reproductive health care:

1. Schools of medicine that train OB-GYN physicians, nurses, midwives, and physician assistants must endorse the legitimacy of trauma, CSA, and posttraumatic stress disorder. They must develop trauma-based interventions within their curricula and ongoing training. By the time medical students participate in clinical experiences, internships, and residencies, the mastery of trauma-informed treatment should be obligatory and measurable.
2. Current providers must gain mastery in identifying, diagnosing, treatment planning, and collaborating across professions to really address CSA in the clinical setting. Provider education should include the goals of raising awareness of CSA survivor rates, disclosure rates, behavioral cues, and the psychological implications of reproductive health care procedures for patients. Further, providers should be trained in effective methods of patient screening for CSA abuse,[24,25] and should include in the standard protocol the "ask early and often" mantra.

3. HCPs need opportunities for clinical supervision that support them through the vicarious traumatization that may occur when working with patients who have significant CSA and trauma history. The Balint method of clinical supervision is an excellent model that addresses the emotional needs and lived experiences of HCPs (http://balint.co.uk/about/the-balint-method/).

4. HCPs should support interdisciplinary, collaborative, components of care through ongoing research with those who interface with CSA survivors, targeting medical students and residents through grand rounds, classroom, and professional consultations with reproductive HCPs to invite across-the-disciplines communications and integrative approaches to patient care.

5. Increase HCP and patient awareness of the long-term effects of CSA through pamphlets and other visual aids prominently displayed in waiting rooms, examination rooms, lavatories, and places frequented by women of childbearing age (eg, pediatric outpatient clinics; Women, Infants, and Children offices; and children's libraries). Media support within the community, through public service announcements, open forums, presentations, and so forth, serve to further disseminate this information.

6. Increase trainings for, and utilization of, specialists in psychosomatic OB/GYN, such as those affiliated with the International Society of Psychosomatic Obstetrics and Gynaecology (see http://www.ispog.org/). HCPs who specialize in psychosomatic OB/GYN are poised to serve the needs of CSA survivor-patients as well as other patients with complex trauma histories. In clinical settings, specialists in psychosomatic OB/GYN can accept at-risk CSA survivor-patients for regular maternity care, just as specialists in preeclampsia accept at-risk maternity patients with high blood pressure. Patients then identify this specialist as their primary OB/GYN provider for seamless prenatal care.

7. Advocate for wellness opportunities in community settings to support awareness of CSA and other trauma survivorship. Support programs that incorporate mind-body integration, such as yoga, for trauma survivors,[26,27] retreats for HCPs who work with CSA survivors, mindfulness-based stress reduction clinics for HCPs, brown bag lunch informational sessions, and so forth. Wellness and integrative health care are excellent options for any community.

8. Support community activities that advocate nonviolence, in particular maternal support programs, sexual assault prevention centers, child abuse prevention programs, and family mentoring programs.

9. Make mental health services more accessible to maternity patients in need, in particular those silently bearing the burden of CSA. Include trauma-trained therapists and social workers in OB/GYN practices. The rationale is clear: maternity care practices see pregnant women more frequently than other medical providers. Mothers who address past CSA and related trauma histories are less likely to become abusive or neglectful parents themselves.[14,17,19] Infants born to mothers who engage in enhancing attachment skills are more likely to become well-adjusted children.[2,4,28] Access to mental health services has a significant ripple effect for the well-being of mothers and infants, families, and communities.

10. Introduce innovative models of pregnancy care that cover multidisciplinary topics, such as the Centering Pregnancy Program.[29] This program is especially helpful for women challenged by socioeconomic stressors and offers an ongoing collaborative relationship between HCPs and patients. Furthermore, Centering Pregnancy programs create opportunities for peer support, partner education, and an ongoing system of natural resources for self-care and family preservation.

Navigating the delicate relationship between providers and patients in reproductive health care is complicated by the unwelcome guest that CSA history becomes for survivors. As caregivers, HCPs have the capacity to respond with compassionate presence, authentic support, and intentional consideration to the most vulnerable patients. It is imperative that providers affirm the dynamic role they play in changing lives through responsible self-care that models the very best practices of what is hoped for CSA survivor-patients.

REFERENCES

1. Ackerson K. Personal influences that affect motivation in pap smear testing among African American women. J Obstet Gynecol Neonatal Nurs 2010;39: 136–46.
2. Ross CA. The trauma model: a solution to the problem of comorbidity in psychiatry. Richardson (TX): Manitou Communications, Inc; 2007.
3. Staples J, Rellini AH, Roberts SP. Avoiding experiences: sexual dysfunction in women with a history of sexual abuse in childhood and adolescence. Arch Sex Behav 2012;41:341–50.
4. Simkin P, Klaus PH. When survivors give birth: understanding and healing the effects of early sexual abuse on childbearing women. Seattle (WA): Classic Day; 2004.
5. Leeners B, Gorres G, Block E, et al. Birth experiences in adult women with a history of childhood sexual abuse. J Psychosom Res 2016;83:27–32.
6. Weinstein AD, Verny TR. The impact of childhood sexual abuse on pregnancy, labor and birth. J Prenat Perinat Psychol Health 2004;18:313–25.
7. Wendt EK, Lidell EA, Westerstahl AKE, et al. Young women's perceptions of being asked questions about sexuality and sexual abuse: a content analysis. Midwifery 2011;27:250–6.
8. Bowen A, Shelley M, Helmes E, et al. Disclosure of traumatic experiences, dissociation, and anxiety in group therapy for posttraumatic stress. Anxiety Stress Coping 2010;43:449–61.
9. Kendall-Tackett KA. Breastfeeding and the sexual abuse survivor. J Hum Lact 1998;14:125–30.
10. Lev-Wiesel R, Chen R, Daphna-Tekoah S, et al. Past traumatic events: are they a risk factor for high-risk pregnancy, delivery complications, and postpartum posttraumatic symptoms? J Womens Health (Larchmt) 2009;18:119–25.
11. Marysko M, Reck C, Mattheis V, et al. History of childhood abuse is accompanied by increased dissociation in young mothers five months postnatally. Psychopathology 2010;43:104–9.
12. Duggal S, Sroufe LA. Recovered memory of childhood sexual trauma: a documented case from a longitudinal study. J Trauma Stress 1998;11:301–21.
13. Seng JS, Sparbel KJH, Low LK, et al. Abuse-related posttraumatic stress and desired maternity care practices: women's perspectives. J Midwifery Womens Health 2002;47:360–70.
14. Klaus P. The impact of childhood sexual abuse on childbearing and breastfeeding: the role of maternity caregivers. Breastfeed Med 2010;5:141–5.
15. Factora-Borchers L, editor. Dear sister: letters from survivors of sexual violence. Oakland (CA): AK Press; 2014.
16. Florian PM. Reproductive health care providers and childhood sexual abuse survivors: minding the gap. Doctoral dissertation. Farmington Hills (MI): ProQuest; 2014.

17. Levine PA. Waking the tiger: healing trauma. Berkeley (CA): North Atlantic Books; 1997.
18. Levine PA. In an unspoken voice: how the body releases trauma and restores goodness. Berkeley (CA): North Atlantic Books; 2010.
19. Van der Kolk BA. Traumatic stress: the overwhelming experience on mind, body, and society. New York: Guilford Press; 2006.
20. Van der Kolk BA. The body keeps the score: brain, mind, and body in the healing of trauma. New York: Viking Press; 2014.
21. Lipskey L. Trauma stewardship: an everyday guide to caring for self while caring for others. San Francisco (CA): Berrett-Koehler Publishers, Inc; 2009.
22. Montgomery E. Feeling safe: a metasynthesis of the maternity care needs of women who were sexually abused in childhood. Birth 2013;40:88–95.
23. Montgomery E, Pope C, Rogers J. A feminist narrative study of the maternity care experiences of women who were sexually abused in childhood. Midwifery 2015; 31:54–60.
24. Kimbrough T, Magyari T, Langenberg P, et al. Mindfulness intervention for child abuse survivors. J Clin Psychol 2010;66(1):17–33.
25. Bernstein DP, Stein JA, Newcomb MD, et al. Development and validation of a brief screening version of the Childhood Trauma Questionnaire. Child Abuse Negl 2003;27:169–90.
26. Emerson D, Hopper E. Overcoming trauma through yoga: reclaiming your body. Berkeley (CA): North Atlantic Books; 2011.
27. West J, Liang B, Spinazzola J. Trauma sensitive yoga as a complementary treatment for posttraumatic stress disorder: a qualitative descriptive analysis. Int J Stress Manag 2017;24(2):173–95.
28. Sperlich M, Seng J. Survivor moms: women's stories of birthing, mothering, and healing after sexual abuse. Eugene (OR): Motherbaby Press; 2008.
29. Massey Z, Rising SS, Ickovics J. Centeringpregnancy group prenatal care: promoting relationship-centered care. J Obstet Gynecol Neonatal Nurs 2006;35: 286–94.

Psychosocial Aspects of Fertility and Assisted Reproductive Technology

Jamie Stanhiser, MD[a],*, Anne Z. Steiner, MD, MPH[b]

KEYWORDS

- Psychosocial • Fertility • Infertility • Assisted reproductive technology (ART)
- Anxiety • Depression • Stress • Mood disorder

KEY POINTS

- Literature evaluating the impact of stress, symptoms of depression and anxiety, and mood disorders on fertility and infertility is limited and inconsistent.
- Stress, symptoms of depression, and antidepressant use may reduce the probability of conceiving for both fertile and infertile women.
- Infertility and miscarriage are associated with considerable psychological burden.
- It is important to screen for stress, depression, and anxiety among infertility patients.

INTRODUCTION

The psychosocial aspects of fertility and assisted reproductive technology (ART) are complex. The extent to which stress, symptoms of anxiety and depression, mood disorders, and psychotropic medication use impact fertility remains unclear. The impact of infertility and ART treatment on psychological well-being, marital and sexual relationships, and the quality of life of couples continues to be researched. The psychosocial implications of ART on our society are considerable and include a shift toward older maternal age, complexities of third-party reproduction, and psychological and socioeconomic barriers to receiving care.

Mood Disorders and Natural Fertility

Stress, anxiety, and depression have significant effects on energy, mood, interests, and self-esteem, all of which may contribute to decreased reproductive efficiency. Depressive symptoms are associated with a 25% to 75% incidence of sexual

Disclosure Statement: The authors have no conflict of interest or disclosures.
[a] Reproductive Endocrinology and Infertility, University of North Carolina, Chapel Hill, NC, USA; [b] Duke University Hospital, 2301 Erwin Road, Durham, NC 27710, USA
* Corresponding author. 7920 ACC Boulevard Suite 300, Raleigh, NC 27617.
E-mail address: jamie_stanhiser@med.unc.edu

dysfunction, including loss of libido, erectile dysfunction, and reduced vaginal lubrication.[1–3] The underlying pathophysiology of the mood disorder may also impact fertility, including disruptions of the hypothalamic–pituitary–adrenal axis, thyroid dysfunction, or hyperprolactinemia.[4] These etiologies can lead to anovulation and reduced fecundity. However, a prospective cohort of 248 ovulatory women enrolled in the Biocycle study failed to find an association between depressive symptoms and reproductive hormone levels or the odds of sporadic anovulation (odds ratio [OR], 1.1; 95% confidence interval [CI], 0.02–5.00).[5] The study was unable to assess the impact of clinical depression on ovulation, because women with history of clinical depression were excluded.

Literature evaluating the impact of psychosocial factors including stress, symptoms of depression and anxiety, and mood disorders on natural fertility is limited and inconsistent. In a prospective, time-to-pregnancy cohort study of 2146 women enrolled in the PRESTO study, Nillni and colleagues[6] found that severe depressive symptoms were associated with decreased fecundability (the probability of conceiving naturally within a given menstrual cycle) compared with no or low depressive symptoms (OR, 0.62; 95% CI, 0.43–0.91). Every 10-unit increase in Major Depression Inventory score was associated with a 10% decrease in fecundability (fecundability ratio, 0.90; 95% CI, 0.83–0.97). In contrast, Lynch and colleagues[7] prospectively analyzed a cohort of 339 women trying to conceive and found no association between self-reported psychosocial stress, anxiety, or depression and fecundability. Interestingly, the authors did find significantly increased fecundability in women reporting higher versus lower social support levels.

The literature on the impact of psychotropic medications on fecundity is also inconclusive. In the PRESTO study, use of psychotropic medications did not seem to decrease fecundability, although a nonsignificant negative trend was noted in current users. Time to Conceive, a prospective, time-to-pregnancy cohort study of 957 women, recently demonstrated a trend toward reduced fecundability with antidepressant use (fecundability ratio, 0.86; 95% CI, 0.63–1.20), which became statistically significant after controlling for history of depression (fecundability ratio, 0.66; 95% CI, 0.45–0.97).[8] These studies suggest that antidepressant use may reduce the probability of conceiving naturally.

Stress and Natural Fertility

The literature suggests that stress and reproduction are interrelated. Psychosocial stress activates the sympathetic nervous system, which may impact the hypothalamic–pituitary–adrenal axis. In the Biocycle study, Schliep and colleagues[9] demonstrated that daily perceived stress interferes with menstrual function. Women with higher daily perceived stress had an increased risk of anovulation and lower luteal phase progesterone levels. Interestingly, baseline stress levels did not predict anovulation, suggesting that it is not chronic stress, but instead daily short-term stressors that affect ovulation.

Biomarkers of stress include corticotrophin-releasing hormone, cortisol, and alpha-amylase.[10,11] Salivary alpha-amylase levels correlate with chronic stress scores and dispositional stress reactivity scores, which measure how a person responds to stressors.[10] Two large prospective studies on preconception stress (the Oxford Conception Study and LIFE Study) found that women in the highest tertile of alpha-amylase experienced a 15% to 29% decrease in fecundability compared with women with levels in the lowest tertile.[12,13] This finding corresponded with a greater than 2-fold increase in the risk of infertility for women in the highest tertile. There was no association with salivary cortisol. Although biomarker levels seem to be associated with fertility, measures of perceived stress (reported by Cohen's Perceived Stress Scale) were not associated with fecundability. Notably, the Perceived Stress Scale is a tool used to measure the perception of stress, not the actual response to stress; Perceived Stress Scale scores do not correlate with alpha-amylase levels.[12]

Psychosocial Factors and Miscarriage

Unfortunately, early pregnancy loss is common, with an estimated 11% to 20% of clinically recognized pregnancies ending in miscarriage. Although most miscarriages are due to chromosomal abnormalities, stress may also play a role. A prospective cohort study of 308 women recruited in early pregnancy found that women who subsequently miscarried had higher corticotrophin-releasing hormone levels and perceived more external demands.[14] Nepomnaschy and colleagues[15] measured daily urinary cortisol levels in the first 3 weeks after conception in 22 women. Women whose cortisol levels increased over baseline were more likely to experience miscarriage. In a Danish population-based study, Bruckner and colleagues[16] conducted a time-series analysis of the Danish unemployment and miscarriage rates. One month after an unexpected increase in the unemployment rate (with consumption of household goods as an indicator of financial insecurity as well), the miscarriage rate significantly increased (β = 33.19; 95% CI, 8.71–67.67). Although this study focused on ambient life stressors, such as economic downturns, other forms of stress seem to increase the risk of miscarriage as well. A recent metaanalysis included studies of psychological stress (measured by structured questionnaires), work stress, life events, health, social support, and perceived stress, and also found that the risk of miscarriage was significantly higher in women exposed to higher levels of these stressors (OR, 1.42; 95% CI, 1.19–1.70).[17] There was significant heterogeneity in the type of psychosocial stress measured, suggesting that a variety of stressors may impact miscarriage risk; however, more research is needed.

Conversely, miscarriage itself can cause significant psychological distress and morbidity.[18] Farren and colleagues[19] prospectively followed 128 women with early pregnancy loss either from miscarriage or ectopic pregnancy and found that 28% met criteria for posttraumatic stress disorder, 32% for anxiety, and 16% for depression at 1 month, and 38%, 20%, and 5%, respectively, at 3 months. In the control group of 58 women with ongoing viable pregnancies, no women met criteria for posttraumatic stress disorder, and 10% met criteria for anxiety and depression. Shapiro and colleagues[20] prospectively followed 1505 pregnant women and found that a history of miscarriage was significantly associated with greater pregnancy anxiety. These findings were confirmed in a recent metaanalysis.[21]

Psychotropic Medications and Miscarriage

Psychotropic medications may also impact the risk of miscarriage. Selective serotonin receptor inhibitors (SSRIs) are the first-line treatment medication for both generalized anxiety disorder and depression. A recent study of infertile women undergoing non-ART treatment found that women on SSRIs did not have an increased risk of first trimester miscarriage; however, non-SSRI medications did increase the risk of miscarriage (relative risk [RR], 1.73; 95% CI, 1.00–3.00).[22] In a nationwide cohort study of all identified pregnancies in Denmark from 1997 to 2010, women exposed to SSRIs during early pregnancy were at an increased risk of miscarriage (hazard ratio [HR], 1.27; 95% CI, 1.22–1.33), as were women who had discontinued SSRI treatment 3 to 12 months before pregnancy (HR, 1.24; 95% CI, 1.18–1.30). The authors concluded that, for women already on SSRIs, continuing treatment would not increase miscarriage risk.[23] Another nationwide cohort study in Denmark from 1996 to 2009 consisting of more than 1 million pregnancies observed that women exposed to SSRI use during pregnancy showed a modest increased risk of miscarriage (HR, 1.08; 95% CI, 1.04–1.13); however, the highest HR for increased risk of miscarriage was among women who had discontinued SSRI use before pregnancy (HR, 1.26; 95% CI, 1.16–1.37).[24] Conversely, in the United Kingdom, Ban and colleagues[25] demonstrated increased risk of miscarriage with SSRI use (relative risk ratio, 1.5; 99% CI, 1.3–1.6), as well as increased risk with non-SSRI use (relative risk ratio, 2.0; 99% CI, 1.7–2.5), and reported a modest increased risk of miscarriage for women who continued with SSRI and non-SSRI medication use in pregnancy compared with those who did not (relative risk ratio, 1.2 [99% CI, 1.0–1.3] and relative risk ratio, [99% CI, 1.5 1.0–2.1], respectively).

Impact of Infertility on Perceived Stress and Mood Disorders

Infertility occurs in 8% to 12% of reproductive-aged couples, and it is nearly universally perceived across society as problematic and distressing.[26] For most couples, the diagnosis and treatment of infertility imposes a significant psychological burden. A study of 200 infertile couples reported that 50% of the women and 15% of the men felt that infertility was the most upsetting experience of their lives.[27] Another study of 488 women concluded that women with infertility felt as anxious or depressed as women who had been diagnosed with cancer, human immunodeficiency virus, or a heart attack.[28]

Many women with infertility have a perceived loss of control over their lives, and experience a sense of loss of identity and feelings of defectiveness.[29] Studies have suggested that hope and personal agency may be important in decreasing psychological symptoms and improving psychological adjustment to infertility.[30]

Depression and anxiety occur in 39% to 41% and 47% of infertile women, respectively, which is twice the rate observed in comparable fertile women.[31,32] Women with a history of recurrent pregnancy loss have quadruple the rate of moderate to severe depression compared with women without a history of pregnancy loss or infertility.[33] Furthermore, ART treatments commonly elevate women's systemic levels of both estrogen and progesterone, which may independently influence mood lability through their actions on serotonin.[34]

Women who seek evaluation and treatment for infertility may be different from women with infertility who do not seek treatment. In a population-based study, Biringer and colleagues[35] retrospectively studied 12,584 Norwegian reproductive-aged women with and without infertility, assessing for anxiety and depressive symptoms using the Hospital Anxiety and Depression Scale. Women with current primary or secondary infertility had levels of anxiety and depression not significantly different from mothers without infertility. However, studies on women undergoing fertility treatment have shown an increased prevalence of anxiety and depressive symptoms compared with population controls.[34]

Impact of Mood Disorders and Stress on the Treatment of Infertility

Infertile women with depression may be less likely to subsequently conceive. First, infertile women who screen positive for depression are less likely to initiate fertility treatments after their initial consultation. Second, fertility treatment in depressed women seems to be less effective. Among infertile women undergoing their first cycle of in vitro fertilization (IVF), those women with a recent diagnosis of anxiety or depression were 40% less likely to conceive (OR, 0.58; 95% CI, 0.41–0.82) compared with women without anxiety or depression.[36] In a national registry of 42,915 ART-treated women in Denmark, a diagnosis of depression before ART treatment initiation was associated with a significantly lower number of treatment cycles and a lower mean number of ART live births compared with women without a diagnosis of depression.[37,38] SSRIs do not seem to impact pregnancy rates after IVF; however; women taking a non-SSRI may have a reduced odds of pregnancy (adjusted OR, 0.41; 95% CI, 0.20–0.80).

Depression may have less effect on outcomes after non-ART fertility treatment. In a secondary analysis of 2 large randomized controlled trials including women with polycystic ovary syndrome or unexplained infertility receiving non-ART therapy (ovulation induction medications with or without intrauterine insemination), symptoms of major depression were not found to impact the probability of live birth.[22]

Although depression is more common among women with infertility, infertile women do not have higher rates of depression as mothers. A cross-sectional study by Salih Joelsson and colleagues[39] compared pregnant women who had conceived with ART with pregnant women who conceived spontaneously, and found no difference in anxiety and depressive symptoms. In a prospective cohort study by Agostini and colleagues,[40] women who had experienced multiple unsuccessful IVF/intracytoplasmic sperm injection cycles had significantly increased anxiety and depression scores during their pregnancy (from 22 weeks of gestation to 15 days after delivery) compared with patients who conceived with their first IVF/intracytoplasmic sperm injection cycle. However, findings from the All Our Babies Study, a prospective cohort study of 1654 pregnant women, suggest that by 4 months postpartum, there is no difference between mothers who conceive using ART and those who conceive spontaneously in the rate of depressive symptoms, anxiety, or perceived stress.[41] Interestingly, first-time mothers who conceived with ART were statistically significantly less likely to report low parenting morale compared with those who conceived spontaneously. This may be due to the highly desired and long-awaited nature of ART pregnancies.

Major depression in the male partner of an infertile couple may negatively affect their probability of success with treatment. In a study by Evans-Hoeker and colleagues,[22] the female partner of a male with symptoms of major depression was less likely to achieve conception (RR, 0.44; 95% CI, 0.20–0.98) and live birth (RR, 0.39; 95% CI, 0.13–1.16). This phenomenon may be because men with depression are more likely to have abnormal semen parameters. In a study of 353 men, depression, as assessed using the World Health Organization (five) Well-Being Index, was associated with decreased sperm concentration.[42] Similarly, Wdowiak and colleagues[43] showed that depression and anxiety resulted in both lower semen volume and sperm concentration.

Impact of Infertility and Assisted Reproductive Technology on the Couple

In addition to its negative effect on psychological well-being, studies have demonstrated that infertility can negatively affect sexual relationships.[44] Evidence is inconclusive regarding the effect of infertility on marital relationships and quality of life.[44] A study comparing fertility-related stress experienced by wives and husbands in infertile couples with other sources of stress experienced by couples without a history of infertility, revealed that higher levels of stress, regardless of whether the stress originated from fertility or another life issue, was associated with impaired marital function and decreased quality of life for both partners.[45] Stress from any source had more impact on the lives of the wives than of the husbands.[46] For wives, fertility-related stress had a stronger negative effect on self-efficacy and sexual identity than did stress from other sources.[46]

Infertility treatment with ART is associated with considerable costs, and this may also have significant psychosocial implications. The national average cost for an IVF cycle is $12,000, before necessary medications, which commonly cost an additional $3000 to $5000. Currently only 15 U.S. states mandate some form of infertility insurance coverage. For patients who do not have insurance coverage or the socioeconomic status and resources to pay for treatment out of pocket, this treatment barrier can be insurmountable. This circumstance can leave couples feeling hopeless and helpless, and biases care toward the socioeconomically privileged.

Sadly, such life stressors may negatively impact ART outcome. A metaanalysis of prospective studies demonstrated a small but statistically significant association between stress and reduced clinical pregnancy rates with ART.[47] A systematic review and metaanalysis of the literature performed by Frederiksen and colleagues[48] suggests that psychosocial interventions, most notably cognitive–behavioral therapy, for infertile couples undergoing ART can reduce psychological distress including depressive symptoms, anxiety, stress, and marital distress (Hedges g, 0.59; 95% CI, 0.38–0.80) and improve clinical pregnancy rates (RR, 2.01; 95% CI, 1.48–2.37).

Because of the pervasive and deleterious nature of stress, depression, and anxiety in couples struggling to conceive, it is important to screen for the presence of these factors in the population of patients with infertility and advocate for psychological evaluation and intervention when appropriate. The potential benefits of such screening and intervention include overall patient well-being, quality of life, compliance with fertility treatments, and enhanced chances of pregnancy. The European Society of Human Reproduction and Embryology has evidence-based guidelines consisting of 120 recommendations for the provision of routine psychosocial care for patients with infertility, which can be accessed at https://www.eshre.eu/guidelines-and-legal/guidelines/psychosocial-care-guideline.aspx.[49]

Societal Shift Toward Advancing Maternal Age

More women in our society are choosing to delay childbearing in deference to pursuing education and developing their careers. National Vital Statistics show that, in the United States, first birth rates continue to decrease for women in their teens, 20s, and early 30s, and are increasing each year for women in their late 30s and 40s. The mean maternal age at first birth in the United States increased from 24.9 to 26.4 years of age from 2000 to 2016, which is a record high for the nation.[50]

Reproductive age beyond 35 years significantly increases a woman's risk for infertility, pregnancy loss, and maternal–fetal medical complications, although these risks are often not realistically portrayed in our culture.[51] Mills and colleagues[52] published, "'Forty is the new twenty': an analysis of British media portrayals of older mothers," and observed that later childbirth in women older than 35 years received extensive media interest, was positively affirmed, and ART was portrayed as a cure for infertility, with disregard for age-related pregnancy risks. The American Society for Reproductive Medicine (ASRM) urges the promotion of a more realistic understanding of maternal age and delayed reproduction, including education on its potential for compromised outcomes and for potential childlessness.[51] Similarly, although treatment with oocyte and embryo donation may improve birth rates for women in their 40s and 50s, the ASRM Ethics Committee discourages the treatment of women over the age of 55 years because of the high risk for pregnancy complications and concerns regarding maternal longevity.[53]

Although it is known that maternal age increases medical and obstetric risks, researchers are now investigating how older maternal age may impact their offspring's socioemotional development. Goisis and colleagues[54] examined 3 large longitudinal birth cohorts consisting of approximately 10,000 children each from the United Kingdom in 1958, 1970, and 2000 to 2002. In each cohort, they assessed the association between maternal age and the offspring's cognitive ability. In the 2 earlier cohorts, a negative association was observed between maternal age and the cognitive scores of the children at 10 and 11 years of age. However, in the most recent cohort, a positive association was observed between maternal age and cognitive scores in the offspring. There were notable differences in the cohorts. In the earlier cohorts, older maternal age was associated with high parity; however, in the 2000 to 2002 cohort older maternal age was associated with higher education and socioeconomic advantage.

Older maternal age in our current society may have benefits for the offspring. Trillingsgaard and Sommer[55] analyzed 4741 families in Denmark and found that older mothers were less likely to use verbal and physical sanctions toward their children, and their children were less likely to have behavioral, social, and emotional problems at ages 7 and 11. These observations persisted when controlling for education level and socioeconomic status. The authors concluded that older mothers seem to thrive better, with improved emotional well-being and psychosocial adaptation. This finding may explain their ability to better tolerate complex emotional stimuli from their children. The authors note, however, that children of women with more support and better health habits do better cognitively.

ELECTIVE OOCYTE CRYOPRESERVATION

Oocyte quality diminishes with advancing age; this phenomenon can lead to pregnancy chromosomal abnormalities, miscarriage, and infertility. Elective oocyte cryopreservation, or egg freezing and banking, is a method of ART used to preserve fertility. Although there are national and clinical level statistics on the success rates with IVF, information on the live birth rates after autologous oocyte preservation is limited to a few published reports including a limited number (<500) of women. Cumulative live birth rates have ranged from 23% to 39%.[56,57]

Success rates do seem to depend on age. In a study of 117 women, Doyle and colleagues[57] modeled the probability of having 1, 2, or 3 children by the number of eggs thawed. To achieve a 70% chance of having at least 1 child, the authors recommend freezing at least 15 to 20 eggs in women less than 38 years of age, and 25 to 30 eggs in women greater than 38 years of age. Unfortunately, older women yield fewer eggs after controlled ovarian hyperstimulation and, therefore, may need multiple cycles to achieve the recommended number of oocytes.

Mesen and colleagues[58] used a decision tree model including natural fertility rates and IVF success rates to determine the optimal age for elective oocyte cryopreservation. The authors modeled oocyte cryopreservation or no preservation at a given age to determine the subsequent probability of a live birth 7 years later. The highest birth rates (70%–90%) were predicted in women who froze their eggs before age 35. The difference in live birth rates between women who freeze or did not freeze their eggs was minimal for ages 25 through 30. However, in the early 30s the difference becomes greater and continues to do so until age 37. According to this model, women who choose to freeze eggs at age 37 have the greatest benefit, with a 50.0% chance of live birth compared with 20.6% chance without freezing eggs.

A recent qualitative study of Dutch women undergoing oocyte banking showed that the majority of women electively freeze and bank their eggs because they are currently unpartnered, and wish to share parenthood with a future partner rather than becoming a single parent.[59] Data from the US National Survey of Family Growth (2006–2010) suggests, however, that as women age their probability of marrying decreases.[60] Women in their 20s are most likely to marry in the next 7 years, whereas women who have not married by age 32, 35, and 39 years have a 30%, 20%, and 10% likelihood of marrying in the next 7 years, respectively. When Mesen and colleagues[58] included marriage rates in their model, they found no benefit to egg freezing at any age. In fact, only 10% of women return to use their eggs; one-half of them have a partner, the other one-half use donor sperm.[56]

Elective oocyte cryopreservation is an expensive solution to a societal issue. The average cost for an egg freezing cycle is $9000, with $500 a year required for storage. Some companies cover a considerable portion of the costs of egg freezing for their female employees; however, this could be encouraging women to delay childbearing in deference to their careers. Despite findings that egg freezing is unlikely to be beneficial for the majority of women, the media, society, and some clinics may mislead women into believing that fertility is guaranteed after banking eggs. The false sense of security and hope that egg freezing offers may prey on women's fears and exploit a vulnerable population. Therefore, the ASRM deems the current evidence on the efficacy, cost effectiveness, and emotional risks of elective egg freezing insufficient to recommend the practice routinely.[61] However, counseling about reproductive aging and the possibility of oocyte cryopreservation should be routine.

Third-Party Reproduction

Third-party reproduction, including gamete (oocyte/egg and sperm) and embryo donation, enables patients with infertility owing to the lack of a male partner or female reproductive ability to conceive. Because of the complex psychosocial issues involved with gamete and embryo donors, recipients, and their offspring, the ASRM strongly recommends psychological evaluation and counseling by a qualified mental health professional before treatment.[62] The psychological assessment should include an interview, with further evaluation as necessary, to rule out any evidence of emotional or financial coercion for all parties.

Before proceeding with treatment as a donor or recipient in third-party reproduction, patients may benefit from psychological counseling to help them navigate the complex emotional and psychological factors involved. These psychosocial factors may become significantly more complex for patients using a known donor compared with the use of an anonymous donor. Counseling for patients undergoing third-party reproduction may include reviewing the potential psychological risks involved, and discussing the positive and negative aspects of disclosing or not disclosing the use of third-party reproduction with the intended offspring. It may also provide the opportunity to address issues of parenting at an older age if applicable, and the possibility of treatment failure. Counseling may also provide psychological skills to aid with processing grief, and help patients to feel peace with the decisions they make.

SUMMARY

The psychosocial implications of infertility ART are considerable. Women's sense of self-identity and personal agency, mental well-being, sexual and marital relationships, reproductive efficiency, compliance with treatment, and pregnancy outcomes are all impacted by these psychological influences. The effects of maternal stress, symptoms of anxiety and depression, mood disorders, and psychotropic medication on fertility and infertility treatment success need further study and understanding. Clinicians need to understand these concerns, screen for, and identify couples struggling with the psychological, emotional, and social aspects of fertility and ART, to best guide their patients' care during their quest to conceive.

REFERENCES

1. Williams K, Reynolds MF. Sexual dysfunction in major depression. CNS Spectr 2006;11(8 Suppl 9):19–23.
2. Fabre LF, Clayton AH, Smith LC, et al. Association of major depression with sexual dysfunction in men. J Neuropsychiatry Clin Neurosci 2013;25(4):308–18.
3. Gelenberg AJ, Dunner DL, Rothschild AJ, et al. Sexual functioning in patients with recurrent major depressive disorder enrolled in the PREVENT study. J Nerv Ment Dis 2013;201(4):266–73.
4. Doyle M, Carballedo A. Infertility and mental health. Adv Psychiatr Treat 2014; 20(5):297. LP-303. Available at: http://apt.rcpsych.org/content/20/5/297.abstract.
5. Prasad A, Schisterman EF, Schliep KC, et al. Depressive symptoms and their relationship with endogenous reproductive hormones and sporadic anovulation in premenopausal women. Ann Epidemiol 2014;24(12):920–4.
6. Nillni YI, Wesselink AK, Gradus JL, et al. Depression, anxiety, and psychotropic medication use and fecundability. Am J Obstet Gynecol 2016;215(4):453.e1-8.
7. Lynch CD, Sundaram R, Buck Louis GM, et al. Are increased levels of self-reported psychosocial stress, anxiety, and depression associated with fecundity? Fertil Steril 2012;98(2):453–8.
8. Casilla-Lennon MM, Meltzer-Brody S, Steiner AZ. The effect of antidepressants on fertility. Am J Obstet Gynecol 2017;215(3):314.e1-5.
9. Schliep KC, Mumford SL, Vladutiu CJ, et al. Perceived stress, reproductive hormones, and ovulatory function: a prospective cohort study. Epidemiology 2015; 26(2):177–84.
10. Nater UM, Rohleder N. Salivary alpha-amylase as a non-invasive biomarker for the sympathetic nervous system: current state of research. Psychoneuroendocrinology 2009;34(4):486–96.
11. Hellhammer DH, Wust S, Kudielka BM. Salivary cortisol as a biomarker in stress research. Psychoneuroendocrinology 2009;34(2):163–71.
12. Lynch CD, Sundaram R, Maisog JM, et al. Preconception stress increases the risk of infertility: results from a couple-based prospective cohort study–the LIFE study. Hum Reprod 2014;29(5):1067–75.
13. Buck Louis GM, Lum KJ, Sundaram R, et al. Stress reduces conception probabilities across the fertile window: evidence in support of relaxation. Fertil Steril 2011; 95(7):2184–9.
14. Arck PC, Rücke M, Rose M, et al. Early risk factors for miscarriage: a prospective cohort study in pregnant women. Reprod Biomed Online 2008;17(1):101–13.
15. Nepomnaschy PA, Welch KB, McConnell DS, et al. Cortisol levels and very early pregnancy loss in humans. Proc Natl Acad Sci U S A 2006;103(10):3938–42.
16. Bruckner TA, Mortensen LH, Catalano RA. Spontaneous pregnancy loss in Denmark following economic downturns. Am J Epidemiol 2016;183(8):701–8.
17. Qu F, Wu Y, Zhu Y-H, et al. The association between psychological stress and miscarriage: a systematic review and meta-analysis. Sci Rep 2017;7(1):1731.
18. Krosch DJ, Shakespeare-Finch J. Grief, traumatic stress, and posttraumatic growth in women who have experienced pregnancy loss. Psychol Trauma 2017;9(4):425–33.

19. Farren J, Jalmbrant M, Ameye L, et al. Post-traumatic stress, anxiety and depression following miscarriage or ectopic pregnancy: a prospective cohort study. BMJ Open 2016;6(11):e011864.

20. Shapiro GD, Seguin JR, Muckle G, et al. Previous pregnancy outcomes and subsequent pregnancy anxiety in a Quebec prospective cohort. J Psychosom Obstet Gynaecol 2017;38(2):121–32.

21. Hunter A, Tussis L, MacBeth A. The presence of anxiety, depression and stress in women and their partners during pregnancies following perinatal loss: a meta-analysis. J Affect Disord 2017;223:153–64.

22. Evans-Hoeker EA, Eisenberg E, Legro RS, et al. Depressive symptoms, antidepressant use, and fertility treatment outcomes. Fertil Steril 2017;108(3):e298–9.

23. Andersen JT, Andersen NL, Horwitz H, et al. Exposure to selective serotonin reuptake inhibitors in early pregnancy and the risk of miscarriage. Obstet Gynecol 2014;124(4):655–61.

24. Johansen RLR, Mortensen LH, Andersen A-MN, et al. Maternal use of selective serotonin reuptake inhibitors and risk of miscarriage - assessing potential biases. Paediatr Perinat Epidemiol 2015;29(1):72–81.

25. Ban L, Tata LJ, West J, et al. Live and non-live pregnancy outcomes among women with depression and anxiety: a population-based study. PLoS One 2012;7(8):e43462.

26. Boivin J, Bunting L, Collins JA, et al. International estimates of infertility prevalence and treatment-seeking: potential need and demand for infertility medical care. Hum Reprod 2007;22(6):1506–12.

27. Potter-Efron P. The Psychological impact of infertility and its treatment. Harv Ment Health Lett 2009;24(11):1–3.

28. Domar AD, Zuttermeister PC, Friedman R. The psychological impact of infertility: a comparison with patients with other medical conditions. J Psychosom Obstet Gynaecol 1993;14(Suppl):45–52.

29. Deka P, Sarma S. Psychological aspects of infertility. Br J Med Pract 2010;3:a336.

30. Omani Samani R, Vesali S, Navid B, et al. Evaluation on hope and psychological symptoms in infertile couples undergoing assisted reproduction treatment. Int J Fertil Steril 2017;11(2):123–9.

31. Hoff HS, Crawford NM, Mersereau JE. Mental health disorders in infertile women: prevalence, perceived effect on fertility, and willingness for treatment for anxiety and depression. Fertil Steril 2017;104(3):e357.

32. Holley SR, Pasch LA, Bleil ME, et al. Prevalence and predictors of major depressive disorder for fertility treatment patients and their partners. Fertil Steril 2015; 103(5):1332–9.

33. Kolte AM, Olsen LR, Mikkelsen EM, et al. Depression and emotional stress is highly prevalent among women with recurrent pregnancy loss. Hum Reprod 2015;30(4):777–82.

34. Williams KE, Marsh WK, Rasgon NL. Mood disorders and fertility in women: a critical review of the literature and implications for future research. Hum Reprod Update 2007;13(6):607–16.

35. Biringer E, Howard LM, Kessler U, et al. Is infertility really associated with higher levels of mental distress in the female population? Results from the North-Trøndelag health study and the medical birth registry of Norway. J Psychosom Obstet Gynecol 2015;36(2):38–45.

36. Cesta CE, Viktorin A, Olsson H, et al. Depression, anxiety, and antidepressant treatment in women: association with in vitro fertilization outcome. Fertil Steril 2016;105(6):1594–602.e3.

37. Sejbaek C, Hageman I, Pinborg A, et al. Incidence of depression and influence of depression on the number of treatment cycles and births in a national cohort of 42 880 women treated with ART. Hum Reprod 2013;28(4):1100–9.

38. Crawford NM, Hoff HS, Mersereau JE. Infertile women who screen positive for depression are less likely to initiate fertility treatments. Hum Reprod 2017;32(3): 582–7.

39. Salih Joelsson L, Tyden T, Wanggren K, et al. Anxiety and depression symptoms among sub-fertile women, women pregnant after infertility treatment, and naturally pregnant women. Eur Psychiatry 2017;45:212–9.

40. Agostini F, Monti F, Paterlini M, et al. Effect of the previous reproductive outcomes in subfertile women after in vitro fertilization (IVF) and/or intracytoplasmic sperm injection (ICSI) treatments on perinatal anxious and depressive symptomatology. J Psychosom Obstet Gynaecol 2017;1–9. https://doi.org/10.1080/0167482X. 2017.1286474.

41. Raguz N, McDonald SW, Metcalfe A, et al. Mental health outcomes of mothers who conceived using fertility treatment. Reprod Health 2014;11(1):19.

42. Zorn B, Auger J, Velikonja V, et al. Psychological factors in male partners of infertile couples: relationship with semen quality and early miscarriage. Int J Androl 2008;31(6):557–64.

43. Wdowiak A, Bień A, Iwanowicz-Palus G, et al. Impact of emotional disorders on semen quality in men treated for infertility. Neuro Endocrinol Lett 2017;38(1): 50–8. Available at: http://europepmc.org/abstract/MED/28456148.

44. Luk BH-K, Loke AY. The Impact of infertility on the psychological well-being, marital relationships, sexual relationships, and quality of life of couples: a systematic review. J Sex Marital Ther 2015;41(6):610–25.

45. Andrews FM, Abbey A, Halman LJ. Is fertility-problem stress different? The dynamics of stress in fertile and infertile couples. Fertil Steril 1992;57(6):1247–53.

46. Awtani M, Mathur K, Shah S, et al. Infertility stress in couples undergoing intrauterine insemination and in vitro fertilization treatments. J Hum Reprod Sci 2017;10(3):221–5.

47. Matthiesen SMS, Frederiksen Y, Ingerslev HJ, et al. Stress, distress and outcome of assisted reproductive technology (ART): a meta-analysis. Hum Reprod 2011; 26(10):2763–76.

48. Frederiksen Y, Farver-Vestergaard I, Skovgård NG, et al. Efficacy of psychosocial interventions for psychological and pregnancy outcomes in infertile women and men: a systematic review and meta-analysis. BMJ Open 2015;5(1):e006592. Available at: http://bmjopen.bmj.com/content/5/1/e006592.abstract.

49. Gameiro S, Boivin J, Dancet E, et al. ESHRE guideline: routine psychosocial care in infertility and medically assisted reproduction—a guide for fertility staff†. Hum Reprod 2015;30(11):2476–85.

50. Martin JA, Hamilton BE, Osterman MJK, et al. National vital statistics reports births : final data for 2013. Natl Vital Stat Rep 2015;64(1):1–104.

51. Sauer MV. Reproduction at an advanced maternal age and maternal health. Fertil Steril 2015;103(5):1136–43.

52. Mills TA, Lavender R, Lavender T. "Forty is the new twenty": an analysis of British media portrayals of older mothers. Sex Reprod Healthc 2015;6(2):88–94.

53. Ethics Committee of the American Society for Reproductive Medicine. Electronic address: ASRM@asrm.org; Ethics Committee of the American Society for Reproductive Medicine. Oocyte or embryo donation to women of advanced reproductive age: an Ethics Committee opinion. Fertil Steril 2016;106(5):e3–7.

54. Goisis A, Schneider DC, Myrskyla M. The reversing association between advanced maternal age and child cognitive ability: evidence from three UK birth cohorts. Int J Epidemiol 2017;46(3):850–9.
55. Trillingsgaard T, Sommer D. Associations between older maternal age, use of sanctions, and children's socio-emotional development through 7, 11, and 15 years. Eur J Dev Psychol 2016;1–15. https://doi.org/10.1080/17405629.2016.1266248.
56. Cobo A, Garcia-Velasco JA, Coello A, et al. Oocyte vitrification as an efficient option for elective fertility preservation. Fertil Steril 2016;105(3):755–64.e8.
57. Doyle JO, Richter KS, Lim J, et al. Successful elective and medically indicated oocyte vitrification and warming for autologous in vitro fertilization, with predicted birth probabilities for fertility preservation according to number of cryopreserved oocytes and age at retrieval. Fertil Steril 2016;105(2):459–66.e2.
58. Mesen TB, Mersereau JE, Kane JB, et al. Optimal timing for elective egg freezing. Fertil Steril 2015;103(6):1551–4.
59. Hodes-Wertz B, Druckenmiller S, Smith M, et al. What do reproductive-age women who undergo oocyte cryopreservation think about the process as a means to preserve fertility? Fertil Steril 2018;100(5):1343–9.e2.
60. Copen CE, Daniels K, Vespa J, et al. First marriages in the united states: data from the 2006 – 2010 national survey of family growth. Natl Health Stat Report 2012;(64):1–22.
61. Practice T, Medicine R, Technology R. Mature oocyte cryopreservation: a guideline. Fertil Steril 2013;99(1):37–43.
62. Practice Committee of American Society for Reproductive Medicine; Practice Committee of Society for Assisted Reproductive Technology. Recommendations for gamete and embryo donation: a committee opinion. Fertil Steril 2013;99(1):47–62.

Moving?

Make sure your subscription moves with you!

To notify us of your new address, find your **Clinics Account Number** (located on your mailing label above your name), and contact customer service at:

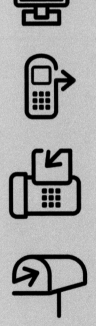

Email: journalscustomerservice-usa@elsevier.com

800-654-2452 (subscribers in the U.S. & Canada)
314-447-8871 (subscribers outside of the U.S. & Canada)

Fax number: 314-447-8029

Elsevier Health Sciences Division
Subscription Customer Service
3251 Riverport Lane
Maryland Heights, MO 63043

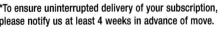